Ayahuasca
Glimpse 2012

Ayahuasca Glimpse 2012

GOITHYJA

Copyright © 2012 by Goithyja.

Library of Congress Control Number: 2012905086
ISBN: Hardcover   978-1-4691-8576-7
             Softcover   978-1-4691-8575-0
             Ebook   978-1-4691-8577-4

The publisher nor the author will be hold responsible by the use of knowledge in this book, the book is intended to educational and spiritual purposes, as adults we make our own choices, so we can not be hold liable by choices made by readers of the book.

All rights reserved. No part of this book may be reproduced or transmitted in any form or by any means, electronic or mechanical, including photocopying, recording, or by any information storage and retrieval system, without permission in writing from the copyright owner.

This book was printed in the United States of America.

To order additional copies of this book, contact:
Xlibris Corporation
1-888-795-4274
www.Xlibris.com
Orders@Xlibris.com

CONTENTS

Introduction		9
Chapter 1	How My Journey Started	15
Chapter 2	Ayahuasca	24
	Conclusion	41
Chapter 3	The Holy Jababa	43
	What is Jababa?	43
	Use among Indians	45
	Jababa Is . .	45
Chapter 4	The Opening of the Third Eye Practical Exercise Eyes of Horus	55
Chapter 5	The Dropping Soma	57
Chapter 6	Maintaining Spiritual Focus	65
Chapter 7	Most Commonly Used Entheogens	154
Chapter 8	Tantra and Shamanism	193
	Similarities	193
	Differences	194
	Tantra	201
	Sexual Ritual	201
	Mantric Practice	205
Chapter 9	Preparation	225
	Balance and Good Humor (Mood)	236
	Experiencing With The Help Of Tantra	237
Bibliography		245

This book is dedicated to my dear and lovely grandmother and to all the light workers who endeavor to accelerate human evolution and help promote peace and love among the dwellers of planet earth; in God we are all sisters and brothers of the universe.

Special thanks to my fiancée, Ana, who supported me all the way to completion of this work also to my brother, friends and people who contribute and help me make possible, the written of this book.

Lord Krishna is every particle manifested in the universe(s); everything who does exist is him! Any other way to interpret God is an illusory, temporal, materialistic way. Experience God and get to know the true meaning of life.

Awakening God within, entheogens & tantra, practical leap to enlightenment.

–Goithyja

INTRODUCTION

Entheogens and Tantra: Awakening God Within, Ayahuasca Glimpse is a book that invites "the dweller of planet earth" to rediscover an enchanted cosmos in the modern world by awakening to the divine within.

The book examines the reemergence of archaic techniques of ecstasy in the modern world by weaving a synthesis of ecological and evolutionary awareness, dance, culture, and the current shamanic reevaluation of entheogenic compounds. Within a narrative framework that enhances consciousness itself to be evolving, the *entheogen* and Tantra emergence of techno-shamanism in the postmodern world that frames the following questions: How can a renewal of ancient initiatory rites arouse and awaken God within? What do trance-dancing expressions speak to in our collective psyche? How do we reinvent ourselves in a disenchanted world dominated by the forces of darkness? (In reality, our egos became stronger than ever.) God never ever withdrew from us; it is impossible because we are part of him. *Entheogen* invites the "dweller of earth" to consider that the answers to these questions lie within the consciousness in each of us and are accessible if only we have the guts and give ourselves permission to awaken to the divine within. Mr. Goithyja is just the real deal, one who truly walks the walk (like in Perceval, for his involvement in the quest of the *Holy Grail*, an allusion to Soma, a ritualistic consecration of it), *and he knows there are many* courageous *people like him out there.* The grail is a symbol of God's grace—available to all, but only fully realized by those who prepare themselves spiritually; it holds the "eucharist" blood of Jesus (soma rasa). *Vedic treatise for extracting soma rasa in present-day research has focused on twenty different plants as "soma," alphabetically mentioned as follows:*

1. *Amanita Muscaria*
2. *Asclepias Acida*
3. *Basella Cordifolia*
4. *Cannabis Sativa*
5. *Ceropegia Decaisneana*
6. *Ceropegia Elegans*
7. *Eleusine Coracana*
8. *Ephedra sp.*
9. *Ichinocarpus Frutescens*
10. *Periploca Aphylla*
11. *Ruta Graveolens*
12. *Sacchaum sp.*
13. *Sarcostemma Acidum*
14. *Sarcostemma Brevistigma*
15. *Sacrostemma Brunonianum*
16. *Sarcostemma Intermedium*
17. *Sarcostemma Viminale*
18. *Sorhum sp.*
19. *Vitis Vinifera (Afgan Grape/Vine)*
20. *Humulus Lupulus (Hops)*

The above list is the outcome of the perception from different schools of thoughts based on the interpretation of Vedic view from their own angle, and it still fails to pinpoint on a plant as soma. *Sarcostemma*, a succulent angiosperm, was supported much by the old school of thought. But *Ephedra*, a gymnosperm enriched with the active drug principle ephedrine, is not a natural habitant of India, where the soma culture existed. The mushroom *Amanita Muscaria*, the latest identified plant as soma, has gained much consensus for its intoxicating and hallucinogenic properties. *Sarcostemma Brevistigma*, is a legendary plant that occupied a significant place in Aryan cult for thousands of years yet remains without any established identification of its integrated original characteristics and ecological niche and still continues to be a botanical enigma.

The soma drinker of ancient India, in reality, knew what soma was about. Soma is more than a bundle of entheogens; soma is the right state of mind and soul achieved by the correct sacramental use of entheogen. The neophyte must take the right dose and have the right mind-set, enhancing the igneous power and vibrating in the exact resonance; only then does the neophyte achieve the soma state. At that moment, he or she experiences God within. So soma is more than plants, fungis, and animal secretions.

The Vedas were passed throughout generations, mostly in verbal mode.

In the beginning . . .

Vyasa got the help of Ganapati for his task. Ganapati writes down the stanzas recited by Vyasa from memory, and thus, the *Mahabharata* is inscribed or written. Ganapati could not cope with Vyasa's speed, and he misses many words and even stanzas.

Upon time, passing on generations, the impure and unholy minds, egos, or "self" of those who deal with such knowledge "veil" some secrets of the holy Vedas, which are being unveiled now, after millennia!.

Goithyja does not believe in miracles. He does know everything in the universe is based on science: *"Knowledge attained through study or practice."*

Many verses from Vedic literature got lost with time, so what we get today is not 100 percent of what was meant to be. This is why sometimes people do not understand the soul of the Vedas.

Most scholars of today cannot cope, and they struggle to identify the true identity of soma mostly because their knowledge is based on temporal illusory physical reality; so their knowledge is not based on the true experimental reality. It is like seeing one side of the coin throughout their whole lives and missing the other!

The purpose of this sui generis book is to guide you and help prepare your mind, body, and soul to endure such spiritual and transcendental journey, leaving behind the dark side of the moon (Maya) or illusory reality, which humankind has embraced.

So we are all trapped in our vests (bodies)—the idea of *unveiling* higher states of consciousness and approach the real states of spiritual enlightenment so advertised in many books but seldom experienced. The teachings in this book were kept in secret for long time. What a labor of giants to unveil such knowledge! Mankind will soon be facing a great degree of purification, cutting our numbers as humans species on earth; our mission is reaching higher vibration and resonance, and we have the opportunity to better experience the universe, which surrounds us in more advanced dimensions of life, "realms" (remember when you die, you keep the same level of consciousness as you were adapted to live on earth, keeping you to experience better reality in the afterlife, keeping you to achieve more advanced spheres in the universe). What does that mean? Don't you think for one second that just going to the church Sunday mornings and listening to what the priest has to say, reading passages of that famous historical book will grant you that awareness; you must work to achieve it. The Lord Jesus did not write one word of that historical book. It does not matter what path you do choose; we must reach the top of the hill. No saint on earth or in the universe will do the job for us. That brings us a question: how bad do we really want it? Remember I am the guy who had the balls to walk the walk. Knowing the way, why not show it? We all live in one world bombarded by materialistic, unreal bull (a world that is crumbling). Do not wait until the last minute to wake up. If you are serious and follow the instructions on this book, you have a real chance to make it. One dive granted by a powerful entheogen like ayahuasca is like reading that historical book for one hundred years! So the experience of the soul is everything; that historical book only gives you speculations!

Being aware that our bodies are made of 100 percent sexual cells, Tantra can help a lot in that endeavor—enhancing in our bodies, minds, and souls the so-called soma states. So what we need to do is just feed our souls a little more. Normally, we keep our bodies fed 24/7, but we do not do the same to our souls; our souls are starving for "practical spiritual knowledge." Tired of theories and fabled tales, many ethnobotanists dedicate their lives to unveil the secrets of soma from the rig Veda ninth mandala, but what they never understood is that we must experience soma to understand what soma is about. Soma is not only a bundle of herbs or fungis; soma is the key to increasing the level of our consciousness. Throughout this book, I do explain what soma is and how to experience it. Jesus tried to explain all that on the consecration of the Holy Grail two thousand years ago, but few understood! Time grabbed that knowledge away from us, and the dark egos of those who control that religion also contribute to that.

Let's talk a little bit more about Goithyja. When I was young, I started seeking better understanding of life–to answer all those familiar questions about who we are, what we are doing here, and where did we all came from. I did not have any religion in my early days until that point. I did not believe in God. (If you are from Rio de Janeiro, Brazil, do you know what I mean?) So when I was introduced to meditation, Transcendental Meditation, and the use of ritualistic entheogen (the plants of light also mentioned by the sutras of Patanjali), I started being inclined to become a believer–plants which bathe our souls with light, "awareness of God within."

What is happening today in our corrupted society, few people on earth really know how to prepare themselves to experience with ritualistic plants of light, actually including fungi on that context. I will try to present in this book a short reference to the science of the Vedas, the importance of spiritual focus, the use of entheogens and Tantra (remember our bodies are made with 100 percent sexual cells–nobody escapes from that reality, even the so-called puritans). Having a brief introduction to those epics, I will explain how important it is to have a path to follow prior, during, and after the whole experience with entheogens (cognitive tools) and Tantra, the importance to keep and save sexual energy, and so on.

In the further chapters, I will explain all that.

CHAPTER 1

How My Journey Started

A long time ago, one friend of mine introduced me to a Brazilian church called Santo Daime, where they offer hoasca tea, or ayahuasca. In Rio de Janeiro, Brazil, the hoasca tea is made of two main plants of light (entheogen). *Ayahuasca,* or "vine of the souls," is an entheogenic potion typically prepared from the liana *Banisteriopsis caapi* and the leaves of the small tree *Psychotria viridis* (also called caapi and yajé, among other names) was explained to me, along with how important it is to prepare our bodies prior to the ritual and doing an external and internal cleanser to having the tea; this sounds weird, but it is very important later on. I learned the importance of preparing our minds, keeping focused to guide us all the way through the whole experience. At the church, they use songs and verses to reach that goal. They call them "hymns." Such songs are received intuitively by the inner voice (which actually is a minor siddhis power). More experienced psychonauts, such as Terence McKenna, advocate taking strong doses, and I totally agree with that idea. Weak doses mean weak experiences; strong doses are more revealing.

The ritual is normally experienced during the nighttime in the weekends far away from big cities and in direct contact with fresh air and lots of trees, starting mostly Fridays. The ritual starts 7:00 p.m. and goes until 4:00 a.m. the next day. Most of the people at the

Brazilian church are advised to wear light white clothes. When the ritual does start, the neophyte is invited to take one glass of hoasca tea, and the dancing follows the celebration.

Later on, I had the opportunity of requesting more information about the "dancing ritual," and it was answered by one of the members of the church. It was explained why when the ritualistic dance starts, we need to suddenly change patterns over and over again. He told me that was necessary to invoke balance between the main powers of the universe—yin and yang. Without that balance of the sexual energy, the experience is not reveling as it should be. The idea is to send the sexual energy to our heads through the Sushumna channel, so I tried to follow up the flux of the flow, and I remember during the dancing ritual, I've the opportunity to stop a couple of times and only have the tea in small cups of glass, sparing one hour from each dose. Long after taking the second dose of the tea, which is by the way very strong indeed, I did notice a sensation on my spinal cord. Suddenly I was fully aware of getting a "boner." So the ritual itself has everything to do with sexual energy. The members of the church try to enforce control over the neophytes; normally they keep the ladies in one side of the court (they try to experience it in a more Christian way, but I do prefer it the Tantra way because it is stronger). After taking the third dose I felt nauseous more and more. I tried hard to avoid throwing up. That was my first contact with that surreal reality, which changed my life forever. During the ritual, again, I suddenly and abruptly felt a strong energy in my spinal cord going straight from my balls to my head; that sensation was repeating itself over and over again. Seconds after that, I had a vision. At the church, members call that vision "miracao." I do believe it was manifesting through the pineal glandule (the third eye). I saw angelic blue humanoid-like entities as seen in the Baghavad Gita. The entities were pouring flowers off a large beautiful vase on my head, attempting to refine and purify my nadis (the channels through and in which, in traditional Indian medicine and spiritual science, the energies of the subtle body are said to flow, and pranayama helps flood our bodies with "prana", also cleansing such channels. Throughout that action, later on, I learned those beings interact in a more refined realm, where they do manifest themselves—entities full of love and knowledge. One of those beings were also bathing my head with some kind of divine solution; when he reached out for my head, I went in a trance state. "Nirvana, samadhi"? At that moment, I had no grasp of time and self; the ego totally dissolved. When I regained consciousness of my surroundings after a couple of minutes, I started to understand the true meaning of life and who in reality we all are. We are just parts of the universe; we are part of God. We don't experience that reality 24/7 because our brains were made to help us interact and perform better in our realm—the third dimensional "illusory reality." Experiencing more in this trapped realm, we do think this is it, and the rest is unreal. In reality, our souls never die but our bodies do (decay). So in one reality, the true one, we do live forever; and in the other, we just live for a couple of years, and that is the truth! At that moment, I've had some kind of revelation: how important it is to re-approach God through meditation. Yes, meditation. Yogis, in the sacred mountains of the Himalayas, can fast for forty days. Can we do that? So how can we go deep into those states of spiritual reality? By the help of entheogen—the ritual which the ancients were pretty aware of. We just lost contact with that reality. All that struggle started when the Roman Catholic Church initiated a widespread killing of shamans by burning them alive, killing their present and past; burning manuscripts of the Mayas, Aztecs, Incas, and many indigenous people; the so infamous and stupid crusades, inquisition, killing millions of people (in present-day count, but thousands many centuries ago; meaning millions today) so as to throw in our heads that crooked religion. They took from mankind the smartest way to reestablish contact within with the creator of the universe, God. More and more, we experience that reality as we come closer to the creator of all, bringing more wisdom to our daily lives. Jesus talked about that on the consecration of the Holy Grail. By the way, he did not write one word on that famous historical book.

Below is a small quotation and tribute to those who die trying to bring the truth to the eyes of mankind:

One of the most difficult pieces of information to find are the names of all the martyrs who were murdered by the Roman Catholic Church down through the ages. Most of them were burned alive—yes, alive! These true Christians were murdered because they loved the scriptures, had portions of *a true* Bible, the true Gnostics, and/or an entire Bible. The believers were hunted down and murdered by the bloodthirsty men of the inquisition, under the direct command of the Catholic Church. Probably no Christian group in history was persecuted more for their beliefs than the Waldensians or the Vaudoix. In the dissemination of the true scriptures and teaching the truth to many in spite of the Roman Catholic inquisition and even prior to the official start of the inquisition *many were murdered*. They were trying to bring to us the true meaning of the *sacramental use of the Holy Grail*. They were the ones who chose to distribute the true Bible based on the manuscripts which were untouched by the Gnostics and Roman Catholics. Many died trying to bring the true scriptures to others. The King James Bible and its history are bathed in the blood of the martyr, and the modern versions are bathed in those who murdered them. *May the Lord open your eyes, once for all,* to the reality of the Bible you treat with contempt based upon what some well-paid seminary professor or pastor states. So the next time you use your modern version, *look for the blood stains on its pages.*

The pouring of divine ether was also to reorganize my main centers of sexual energy, chakras (the Vedas explains all that), the whole experience was strong. I could be taking one more dose of the hoasca tea but I felt very nauseated; so to avoid throwing up, I decided to stop (each dose is around sixty milliliters of the very strong tea). I understood how important it is to have a spiritual path to follow up. Later on, talking to members of the Brazilian church, I noticed most of them take only small doses of the tea to avoid getting nauseated. Sacrificing with that action, so the whole experience is weak. We did experience something like the one described by Audous Huxley in his book, *The Doors of Perception,* by seeing supernaturally brilliant colors, making the percipient aware of fine shades and landscapes. It does not matter which entheogen was taken—weak is weak! I went really deep by pure luck because I did not have had any prior experience with hoasca tea; so, at that moment, I did not know the hassle of getting nauseated, by taking the hoasca tea, the nausea effect stops most of the people into having a more profound spiritual experience. By not taking strong doses anymore, like the Terence McKenna advocates, they reduce the opportunities to go deep within; the whole experience is compromised. It is like smoking one little joint, you can't go deep. Go strong or don't waste your time, strong but under control, not over. By the way, the ritualistic experiences are done between fifteen days to let the "disciple" or "psychonaut" rest his or her body quite well because that stuff is hard in our digestive systems. By 3:30 a.m. the ritual was getting to the end, so I started gaining more awareness of our realm—the three-dimensional one. After that, my fiancée and I left the Brazilian church around 5:00 a.m. My fiancée, Ana, drove the car back home. When we arrived, we took a nice shower and lay to rest, getting some sleep. During the sleep, I started having an amazing experience. I felt like leaving my body and going to some place, on a vivid dreamlike experience. It was pretty lucid all the way. In the vivid dream, I met with the founder of the Brazilian church who just passed away a couple of years before; he was gathering others members of the Brazilian church in the spiritual realm, some kind of farm surrounded by beautiful trees and incredible sharp clear images of everything who I looked at. The whole experience opened my eyes to understanding how important it is to overcome our fears. Not only that but by having immense power of concentration (focus), we can control much better the whole experience. You cannot blink your eyes; if you do so, you are automatically transported back or to another place. So focus is the key, and Tratak helps us achieve that mental acuity.

I understood that all of that has got to do with opening the third eye, which is imperative to have a nice spiritual experience. This is why it is so important to prepare mind, body, and soul prior to the experience. If we don't do that, we can end up being trapped inside our *subconscious* minds having only vivid thoughts influenced by our own minds (like vivid hallucinations). That is the difference between a useful spiritual awareness and just a waste of time! When the body and mind is not clean enough, blocks of stress accumulated in our minds do start influencing and generating the so-called *bad trip.* So if you have bad thoughts, you will create vivid images in your own mind ruining the whole experience. By keeping your mind clean and focused on spiritual thoughts, you guide your soul to more profitable experiences; the fear is due to the incompatibility between man's egotism and the divine purity between man's separateness of God within. The disciple, or psychonaut, seeing only colorless and subtly shifting hallucinations of emotional, complex patterns like Persian carpets and bizarre landscapes easily seen in the darkness, or when your eyes are closed, is like wasting her or his time. Unveil the secrets of other realms and let it change your life for the better.

At that day, I felt like having the privilege to experience higher states of consciousness; and I cannot deny passing through my mind thoughts of all those guys who go to conventional churches to listen of priests talking about God but never ever experiencing God. So when they do feel something, mostly in Baptist churches, the feeling is influenced by the hard work of spiritual light workers, working in their clogged chakras, releasing blocks of stress. Because sure is better than nothing *but not good enough nor deep enough to transform us.* So trying to describe some mystic religious experience is like trying to explain the taste of a rare, not well-known fruit only found deep inside the Amazon jungle. I can try and spend hours trying to describe the taste of that amazing fruit, but in reality, you will never know for sure. Only those who have the experience and "walk the walk" know for sure.

Why is that so important?

To experience a much better existence in more purified realms of existence, we must expand our consciousness approaching more and more to that reality and diving within to become more and more enlightened, until the day we do burn our egos completely—that is *enlightenment* pure and clear. Why not? Who wants to live in a gross realm like our own forever? Seven billion people will not last; our planet cannot sustain for long period of time all that people dumping, eating, polluting, etc. The reorganization process is already set on and will get nasty pretty soon. But there is hope to those who in time understood the true meaning of life. If you did not get the picture yet, pretty soon you will. My sincere wishes is to more and more people achieve higher levels of consciousness and experience God, and the key to reach that reality is through the use of entheogen, meditation, and *love*. Entheogen is a quantum leap for that reality, a personal-growth experience, which often occur in the form of a quantum leap—a strong and radical shift from one mind-set to another. There may be a number of small steps leading up to that leap, but at some point, there is a big change, and it happens in an instant. Most of the time, when people pursue personal growth, they simply don't invest enough time and energy in a consistent direction to achieve a quantum leap. Maybe you've read a book on getting organized, and while you were reading it, the positive energy you experienced moved you closer to making a leap. You felt fairly certain at the time that this was going to work. But then you finished the book (or got sidetracked and didn't finish it*)*, and the impact of the book gradually faded. You never reached the quantum leap that allowed you to break through to a new level of order in your life. Over a period of days or weeks, your old pattern reasserted itself. Sounds familiar? So what does work? How do you achieve a quantum leap? Why must the entheogenic dose as emphasized by Terence McKenna be strong? You need to exert some effort in a particular direction where you want to grow, and you need to consistently sustain it until you achieve a quantum leap. If you stop short, you'll likely fall right back to where you started. So first of all, if you're going to target a new quantum leap, you need to commit to sustaining that effort until you hit the leap.

This is why I say personal growth is very hard. Achieving a quantum leap is tough work. It requires a strong force of sustained effort, and you can't let up until you hit the leap. If you get sidetracked for too long, you have to start over again.

Soon I will talk about Jababa, the real achievable quantum leap to most people who try entheogens and are pretty familiar with ayahuasca tea. They already know the importance of strong doses, but in steps with caution. But what about the fabled secretive oo-koo-he? And what about Jababa? Why Jababa? I sought during many years, one way or another, to experience higher levels of consciousness using entheogens without throwing up or being nauseated, and Jababa is the answer for all that. In the next chapters, I would talk little bit more about ayahuasca tea and why, in the end, my option points toward Jababa—the secretive entheogen from the Brazilian Amazon jungle.

CHAPTER 2

Ayahuasca

Ayahuasca (meaning *vine of the souls* in Quechua) is an entheogenic potion typically prepared from the liana *Banisteriopsis caapi* and the leaves of the small tree *psychotria viridis* (also called caapi and yajé among other names). Traditional ayahuasca use is widespread in South America, having been reported in Venezuela, Colombia, Panama, Brazil, Peru, Ecuador, and Bolivia. No less than seventy-two indigenous groups are reported to have used entheogenic ayahuasca potions, and there are forty-two different indigenous names for the potions. Archaeological research has shown that the use of ayahuasca in Ecuador dates back as many as five millennia. Normally, the ayahuasca brew is ingested orally, usually in a shamanic or ethno-medicinal context. Ayahuasca visions are an important component of Amazonian art. The visionary experience of *ayahuasca* is so important and fundamental to the world view of the Amazonian Indians that the use of the potion by *cure(a)nderos* has largely survived the forces of acculturation; and metizos consult the *ayahuasca* plant teachers even in modern-day cities.

The base of the ayahuasca brew, *Banisteriopsis caapi*, contains the betacarboline alkaloids harmine and harmaline, the same alkaloids found in the Syrian rue *Peganum harma-la*. Indeed, these alkaloids are widespread, having been found in well over one hundred species in more than twenty-seven families representing more than sixty genera. More than ninety different plant species from thrity-eight plant families have been reported as *ayahuasca* admixture. The admixture plants may be categorized into the three broad categories: therapeutic, stimulants, and entheogenic or visionary additives. The last category may be divided into four broad subcategories: *nicotiana* (nicotine); *brugmansia* (tropane alkaloids); *brunfelsia* (scopoletine); and *chacruna/chagropanga* (DMT). All of these plants have the same pharmacological purpose in *ayahuasca*—to enhance the entheogenic/visionary quality of the potions as an aid to shamanic divination. All of the plants in the first three subcategories are members of the family Solanaceae, whereas the tryptamine-containing category involves plants in the families Malpighiaceae and Rubiaceae. The most common *ayahuasca* admixture plant in use in Amazonian Peru, also used in Amazonian Ecuador and *Brazil*, is *psychotria viridis*. It is known as *chacruna* in Peru and *samiruca* or *amirucapanga* in Ecuador. The leaves of this shrub are added to the *ayahuasca* brew to strengthen its entheogenic potency. The short term MAO inhibiting property of the betacarbolines allows the normally orally inactive DMT to be orally active, producing the entheogenic effects of the potion. The pharmacological principles of the *ayahuasca* potion are present in many plants throughout the world, not just limited to South America. By combining these plants in appropriate combinations, several thousand ayahuasca-like potions are possible.

Why is it that in most countries entheogens are outlawed? It is the dark side working against mankind's awareness of God within! So let us awake God consciousness before it is too late. Nobody has the right to create stupid laws to avoid man from seeking his true identity! That kind of behavior is mostly common among materialistic guided countries, which urges us to tamper with and into the true nature of human freedom; an individual must have the right to do whatever he/she wants with his/her own body without the authoritarian interference of the government. In the United States, they talk a lot about freedom; in reality, it just theoretical talks. Most entheogens in North America are outlawed.

It is useful at the outset of this discussion to mention our shared culture of dishonesty. We have all been dishonest or infected by someone else's dishonesty regarding the use of drugs. The term "drugs" is taken lightly because it symbolizes in a word our shared self-deception regarding a set of substances which are randomly classified on one basis or another. A substance has a powerful effect on the mind or body. It may change desires or experiences. It generally alters neurochemistry, causing symptoms typical of addiction. In other words, we determine what substances will or will not be classified as drugs on the basis of what their effect on the mind and body, not on the basis of what they actually *are*. Furthermore, a substance may have addictive side effects, but if these do not lead to clinically significant impairment, then it is considered benign enough to even be sold in our markets such as alcohol and tobacco. The point is that society's opinion of drugs is a *reaction to effects* more than anything else. What does this have to do with dishonesty and how is that relevant to a discussion of psychedelics? Firstly, the notion of a substance being a "drug" means that it is psychologically classed as a hazard with all the religious, social, legal, and political stigmas associated with drug abuse. It means the first notion of individuals is to react mentally with these negative associations. Of course, this is deceiving because it muddles the reality that drugs serve so many essential and productive functions in society such as in medicine. However, in the case of psychedelics, people tend to immediately conjure up prejudices regarding drug use in the 1960s onward as an expression of youthful rebellion. So psychedelics have become synonymous with rebellion and anarchy in the public mind. This psychological prejudice also includes the false impression that somehow this American phenomenon interweaving psychedelics and youthful rebellion is somehow a universal truth not worth questioning or revisiting. Given such a climate of suspicion and self-certainty, what are the chances that *shamanistic traditions* would ever be weighed with due process culturally, legally, and academically? Shamanistic traditions are suspect as foreign oddities to begin with, but the added fact that they make regular use of psychedelic drugs makes them especially anathema. But then, shamans do not use the word "drug," nor are they encapsulated in a lifestyle of Western stigmas. They do not use drugs at all in our sense. In fact, the closest rendering in English to what they are using is "entheogen," which roughly translated means "creating the god within," and they have been doing it for thousands of years without destroying society, without Western values, and with some remarkably positive social results. Irony would have it that eventually Western society would reconsider its positions on ancient traditions beyond which we have thought ourselves to have "evolved." Furthermore, that irony is carried into the realm of drugs precisely because these lesser "backward" societies have appeared to have found positive uses for psychedelics, which our "advanced" society has not and which must serve as a bitter reminder of our failure to do what we do best: profit from nature. In reality, the idea is to highlight changing American trends in the realm of psychedelics. Shamanistic redemption as a form of entheogenic intervention with drug abusers is discussed as a treatment option. There are three significant trends which have developed in the domain of subjects surrounding psychoactive drugs. Perhaps, most dramatically, a trend of judicial tolerance for the religious use of psychoactive drugs listed as controlled substances has solidified up to the high levels of the legal system. There is also an academic trend of renewed research interest into reexamining the properties of psychoactive drugs for clinical use in therapy. Finally, there is a cultural trend of dissatisfaction with Western values and a search for a more eclectic existentialism which is tied to ancient sources of wisdom and a deep regard for the holistic importance of balance within nature. Psychedelic entheogens are used to achieve prophetic insight into the Western impoverishment in naked and rampant capitalism which enslaves the minds of humankind while destroying the environment. Each of these trends will be discussed in further chapters of the book, but it must be noted that hints of each trend will be woven into the accounts of the others blurring at times the distinction between categorizing these human phenomena. For example, through judgment and enforcement, the law influences cultural development. Cultural trends can sway legal interpretations and sentiments. Research informs the law and culture. The law can bind or open the doors for research. Culture can generate interest in novel research. This is what will be seen in the following critique as the trends have worked together to provide a new context for a distinct era in drug use as entheogens that can liberate addicts and open up new inner worlds for safe spiritual exploration. Drug use is old, and its purposes are many. The most misunderstood of these purposes, as indicated by the scientific, religious, and political establishments' suspicions, has been the use psychedelic substances to achieve spiritual enlightenment. These suspicions are not difficult to understand on the surface given the categorization of psychedelic drugs as hallucinogens. Hallucinogens are defined by the U.S. government as substances which alter a person's perception of reality to the extent that persons. It is therefore quite reasonable that government employees charged with writing, interpreting, and enforcing the laws be confident that they can hold citizens to these standards in the same reality as their own. In other words, this faith in a universally shared reality has to be the foundation of any functional society. And yet, the social problems with psychedelics go further than harmless dissociations and daydreaming because of the intensity of hallucinogenic experiences which impairs reasoning and judgment in simple tasks such as driving a car or lighting a match. However, when examined through a cultural and historical lens, this negative and antisocial legal stigma placed on psychedelics is a Euro-American phenomenon which has recently been highlighted in the case of one notable psychedelic: ayahuasca. The background of use of ayahausca or hoasca tea by a contemporary religious group, the Uniao do Vegetal (UDV) the group has around eleven thousand members and one hundred communities in Brazil and abroad. The UDV uses hoasca as a religious sacrament made of two plants, *Banisteriopsis caapi* (mariri or jagube) and *Psychotria viridis* (chacrona or rainha). Psychotria viridis contains the controlled substance N, N-dimethyltryptamine (DMT) (Bullis, 2008): the active ingredient in *Banisteriopsis caapi,* which "protects the DMT from being deactivated by gastric enzymes" so that DMT can be effectively taken orally. Hoasca is ingested twice a month by the members, including small amounts by pregnant women and adolescents, with no adverse affects. In contrast to the Western view of altered states of consciousness as promoting "alienation, excessive introspection, rebelliousness as well as illegal behaviors," the UDV uses hoasca tea as a hallucinogenic decoction in rituals of "spiritual, emotional, and ethical support." The Brazilian government has granted legal permission for the use of hoasca in religious ceremonies. Formal research was also undertaken in 1993 to provide data on the psychopharmacology of hoasca for safe consumption. Psychological profiles of long-term members showed healthier personalities and superior neuropsychological functioning when compared to normal controls. European explorers in Mesoamerica considered equated the use of hoasca with worshipping the devil, and missionaries used their force to repress "traditional religious beliefs and practices in order to save the native peoples by obliging them to abandon customary practices and embrace the Christian faith." These actions did unchain a wide killing spree of shamans in the Americas; actually, this forced the natives into various syncretistic religious systems which blended Christian beliefs and indigenous cosmologies. The UDV mingles elements of Christianity with shamanism and spiritism. Shamans value altered states of consciousness as a means to interacting with spirits and forces of nature. Hoasca induces members to have a shamanic experience. In this spiritual realm, it has been used to "obtain divine guidance and to communicate with the spirits that animate the plants; to achieve trance states; to train prospective shamans; to induce dreams so as to divine the future; for prophecy; as a telepathic agent; to cure illness through psychic or physical means; as a preventive agent against the malice of other people; as a diagnostic tool where the visions are used to prescribe remedies for illness; to identify an evil doer or agent responsible for illness; and to achieve ecstasy in the service of health and political acumen. In such a diversity of purposes there is a wide range of misunderstandings in diagnosis and treatment that could arise as therapists come into contact with ceremonial hoasca users. The dramatically divergent perceptions of psychedelics of Western society from those of the UDV can be perhaps be understood in the context of the historical debate over psychedelics in the United States from the 1960s when the youth were encouraged by drug culture figureheads, such as Timothy Leary, to reject the older generation's apprehension with drugs and pursue a "better" life through experimentation into mind alteration. Therefore, psychedelics became synonymous in the American mind with youths, a rebellion and recklessness so distinct from the UDV-controlled administration of hoasca to their youths. Consequently, while hoasca has been used beneficially for more than two millennia, further research into it's the therapeutic powers of psychedelics was curtailed due to their unpopularity in the United States. At the psychological level, the general U.S. population is not open to the idea that psychedelics can be life enhancing, positively spiritual, or healthfully imbibed. It is simple incomprehensible, though entirely unverified. In 1999, U.S. government officials seized a shipment of hoasca bound for the UDV by virtue of the Controlled Substances Act (CSA 2000), which lists DMT as a prohibited compound. The church sued for their First Amendment rights. The federal district and federal circuit courts, and the U.S. Supreme Court all ruled in favor of the UDV. Government attorneys argue the government's compelling interests to protect UDV members and prevent the diversion of the sacrament for recreational purposes. The UDV countered by appealing to the Religious Freedom Restoration Act (RFRA 1993) and the exception of peyote that has already been granted for the Native American Church. The government could not provide superior evidence of the risks of diversion for nonreligious use or meet the burden to prove with specific evidence of hoasca's harm. In the case of the previous exemption of peyote for the Native American Church, "there is no dispute that the exemption granted to the Native American Church has been a success, neither producing harmful effects on members nor provoking diverted use among nonmembers of the church. However, it all begs the question why one religion would be protected and just any religion declaring itself to use a controlled substance. In *U.S. v. Meyers* (1995: 1502-03), Michael Myers was arrested for the "intent to distribute and conspiracy to possess marijuana." Another arbitrary action, outlaw such divine plant, "tree of knowledge mentioned on the Bible sharing such place with Iboga tree", He defended himself by claiming that he was the "Reverend of the Church of Marijuana" and that his religion required him "to use and grow marijuana for the good of humankind and the planet earth." On appeal, the court provided a set of criteria in distinguishing sincere religious use from personal philosophies. "Ultimate ideas: They address fundamental questions about the meaning and purpose of life. Metaphysical beliefs: These beliefs are not only fundamental, but must be transcendental. Moral and ethical systems: Religion proposes a system or organized moral and ethical codes. Comprehensiveness of beliefs: These beliefs are also encyclopedic and reach a broad array of issues. The accoutrements of religion: These include a founder or prophet, sacred writings, specified gathering places, keepers of knowledge [ministers, clergy] ceremonies and rituals and holidays." These criteria can be significant in the mental health field as they provide a means for professionals to distinguish sincere religious psychedelic pursuits from drug abuse. These guidelines are also an excellent example of the court's use of the cultural standards of religion to interpret and apply the law. The case also brought out important points regarding our evaluations of others who use hoasca. The government's position is paternalistic in its use of the terms "hallucinogen" or "drug" in that it denigrates its religious character. The brief asserts that the very term "hallucination" carries the implication that the insights gained in such ceremonies are delusionary and false. In other words, as the debate is currently framed in public policy, the government has already established evidence of its own prejudice against shamanistic traditions because the terms are negatively value-laden. Therapists could instead use other terms in these religious contexts, such as "entheogen," "sacrament," or "agent of revelation." The Latin roots of the word "entheogen" translate to mean "in god creates," or in other words, the entheogen creates the god within us or "to become divine within" (Wells, 2007, p. 35), which is substantively more salutary than the term "drug" and nearer to the self-understanding of shamans. Anticipates that organizations appealing for an entheogenic exception will have a profile showing they are an actual religion, have a record entheogenic use, use the entheogen as a central religious requirement, control for risks of recreational diversion of their entheogen, and use the entheogen in sacramental doses that do little or no harm. This legal trend not only validates the cultural trend on entheogenic-based religions, but growing research interests in entheogens. Examine the potential use of hallucinogens such as ayahuasca, ibogaine, or peyote in a redemptive model of drug substitution. "The redemptive model posits that the proper use of one psychoactive substance within a spiritual or clinical context helps free an individual from the adverse effects of their addiction to another substance and thus restores them as functioning members of their community or group." The UDV is examined as an example of a model context in which supportive drug substitution can occur through the use of ayahuasca as the mediating agent. Hallucinogens as drug substitutes are appealing because they do not in themselves cause physical dependence and have successfully been substituted for heroin, alcohol, and methamphetamines. This form of redemption can be both secular and religious and considers many cross cultural perspectives of redemption. It combines the best of Western science with the best of various shamanic traditions to treat addictions. Brazil and Peru, including part of the Amazon, is the origin of ayahausca as it has been used for more than two millennia. Brazil provides a potential example of how cultural attitudes toward hallucinogens can develop over a long period and how they become acceptable in mainstream society, an ethnographic study profiling ecstasy users who attend night clubs and rave parties. They combined information from observational studies, key informants, and interviews with Ecstasy users in Sao Paulo, Brazil. The users were upper class, well educated, and had access to the labor market. Two groups were identified based on the period of their initiation into drug use being at the end of the 1990s when rave parties emerged or in the early 1990s which consisted of more experience users. Neither group had sought help for addiction and both groups had positive beliefs regard safe drug use. Ecstasy has the effect of elevating self-confidence and fosters impulsivity with the illusion of control. Several of the subjects of the study reported driving their cars and having sex at times without condoms. The importance of the study is that it provides a profile of prospective clients who have a desire to use hallucinogens, but need to consider all the risks and alternative approaches to these experiences such as in the UDV. The research value of pointing out the findings is that provides a basis for understanding the very populations which may be rich sources of clients who would be willing to explore an intervention which provides euphoria without withdrawal. Imagine a substance that could give you the insights and visions you seek that would be legal and safe. The hypotheses of such an approach could also help to sort through the diagnostic process particularly with the dually diagnosed. Shamanistic interventions with clients who are foremost addicts may have distinct appeal in contrast with those clients who are foremost mentally ill. In this way, the intervention can be tailored more to treat withdrawal or emotional disturbance. Wells traces the relative nature of different cultural attitudes toward drugs across time. There are few, if any, societies that have not considered at least one drug as acceptable. Research has shown evidence that mushroom inebriation may have been a common practice as long ago as 6000 BC. One researcher even suggested that psychedelic was what first inspired primitive man with the idea of God. In spite of the fact that beginning in 1965, psychedelics became criminal.

    Shamanism has remained a spiritual fixture of the modern world. "Churches that employ psychoactive plants as their sacrament are gaining converts, and traveling to the Amazon to drink hallucinogenic beverages with a spiritual guide has become the fashionable way to holiday for new neo-pagans, adventurers and so-called psychonauts (explorers of inner space)." Research supporting the psychedelic renaissance indicates that psilocybin" can evoke experiences similar to spontaneously occurring mystical experiences, when given in a supportive environment." Terence McKenna, spokesmen for the psychedelic movement, is credited with coining the term "archaic revival" to describe this new wave of entheogenic aficionados. It has been these spiritual pioneers in the context of government control that has spurred the "rise of the entheogenic church "as a "controlled environment for entheogenic exploration." Throughout history and across cultures there has been a universal human tendency to use psychedelic substances to have religious experiences and gain spiritual insight. The meaning of ayahuasca glimpse book is show the right approach towards partaking with entheogenic substances avoiding troubles, However, restrictions in modern society have pushed these experiences into a cultural underground in which individuals are largely left to themselves as to how to organize their experience and integrate their insights. This contrasts with many cultures in the past which developed comprehensive frameworks for the use and benefits of psychedelics. Baker explores the nature of the psychedelic substance as a sacrament in contrast to other purposes with the intent to promote "individually constructive and socially integrative experiences" In an interview between an expert journalist on the Brazilian Amazon and an urban shaman, Machado, who uses hoasca in healing ceremonies, Machado discusses the current trend of drug tourism in which urban Brazilians and Peruvians provide tours including mystical drug experiences. The shaman describes the distinctions between genuine folklore shamanism and the vogue drug tourism. There is currently a spiritual and psychological crisis in Europe and North America precipitating in these quests to resolve personal problems. Machado also discusses the dangers of plant mixtures which include toxins. He is particularly critical of charlatans who fraudulently practice shamanism but "who are liars and cheats and who don't have the capacity, the preparation, or the boldness to do the work." In other words, shamanism is not sponge bath experience. It is hard work. It requires preparation. Some have concluded that the Western spiritual exodus toward shamanism is merely a symptom of boredom and the pursuit of a new entertainment. Drug tourists are charged with being too ignorant of native tribes to understand the nature of real spiritual healing. This may not be true of all people visiting Amazonia or of the guides they employ. In fact, notes the recent case of a bona fide healer, Maria Sabina, who was forced by others to providing healing services to tourists on the threat of having her family killed, It is to question this negative stereotype of these entheogenic pilgrims and to analyze the basis for this phenomenon of Westerners seeking out traditional spiritual treatments including entheogens. One reason why the logic of criticism fails is the lengths to which an addict would have to go to reach Amazonia as well as the nature of the ceremony involving violent vomiting followed by diarrhea and terrifying visions (this occurs when proper previous preparation is neglected by the neophyte). In other words, there is another cultural force at work in the background, a cosmic yearning of which these spiritual pilgrimages is one indication. There is a human need which Western society is not fulfilling but shamanism is, most of western religion is based in mental speculations not in practical experience, the human soul must experience to believe. How does one bind entheogenic research and the Western cultural deficit into one paradigm? *McKenna* has spent over three decades studying the botany, chemistry, and pharmacology of ayahuasca. Through the work of many scientists including McKenna, the ayahuasca has become the most thoroughly researched hallucinogen used by traditional shamans. The plant species used in the preparation of ayahuasca are now firmly understood, including the active ingredients as well as their synergistic properties. Potential healing applications of the entheogen have also been identified. Ayahuascan studies have become a window into "the sacred cosmology of magic, witchcraft, transcendent experience, and healing that permeates and defines the practices of "Pajelanca, ethnomedicine." The current global appeal of the UDV religion lies in its medicinal value to the mind, body, and spirit. McKenna, understands ayahuasca to have a presence of its own, which it is now choosing to assert into human awareness as a messenger to the world regarding a number of unhealthy patterns including rapacious governments, fanatical fundamentalism, consumerism, mindless entertainment, decadent distractions,Hollywood studios spend billions of dollars producing violent garbage every year and throwing all that in our minds, negatively influencing human behavior in, and the frantic but ultimately meaningless pursuits of a civilization that has lost its compass. Ayahuasca is an ancient antidote for the modern, unsustainable "death culture." The implications are that therapists need to reevaluate the assumptions of Western values, because it is their ethical duty to look outside of their values, and this is not just at the individual level. Western society, as a whole, needs to be reevaluated. If the "rapaciousness" of our pursuits turns out to be a root cause of our general pathology, then it behooves our own psychic cause to alter our course. Maybe in the long run there are better, more ancient ways of being social creatures. If we are really committed, sincerely committed to our clients' mental health, then we have to be willing to consider what is really the best for them *in spite of what we might wish was best for them—shamanism and entheogenic intervention.* For millennia, traditional groups have been using certain substances within their communities to fulfill fundamental human needs. Some of these naturally occurring substances have psychedelic properties which are so potent they have ability to mediate the withdrawal from other drugs. At the same time, they are used within a religious context which generates social stability and cohesiveness. However, Western society has yet to consider them as clinical resources for treating addicts in spite of their successful use for thousands of years. A shamanistic intervention using hallucinogens with addicts can provide four options both secular and religious: ayahuasca, ibogaine (is used to cure addiction on heroin), peyote, or LSD. The underlying concept of treatment is that of redemption. Redemption here is not limited to the Christian or any other religious sense. The redemptive model simply put is the "proper use of one hallucinogenic substance within a spiritual or clinical context helps to free an individual from the adverse effects of their addiction to another substance and thus restores them to functioning members of their community or group." So there are two goals of the intervention: (1) free the individual from addiction, and (2) reintegrate the addict into society as a functioning member. Two mechanisms operate in the intervention to spur change. First, there is the psychological element of suggestibility which means the learning process by which the individual pursues abstinence from alcohol and opiates as a way of life. Second, there are neurophysiological and neurochemical properties of the hallucinogens which are the subjects of ongoing research for their ability to "obviate and negate the cravings for and withdrawal effects" of drugs. Furthermore, these hallucinogens are fascinating in and of themselves because they do not cause physical dependence and have more recently been used to mediate withdrawal from heroin, alcohol, methamphetamines, and other drugs. These redemptive hallucinogens are ayahuasca (used in a drink of *Banisteriopsis caapi* and *Psychotria viridis* mixed together), *ibogaine (from Tabernanthe iboga)*, LSD (derived from the fungus *Claviceps purpurea*), and peyote (*Lophophora williamsii*). Also, unlike other drugs which induce memory loss, these substances heighten and shift perceptions, thoughts, and feelings while maintaining complete memory and total consciousness of the user. In the case of these traditional societies, it is helpful to further explain the details of suggestibility. The hallucinogens themselves have the power to place users in a suggestible state in the sense that ideas and narratives will be introduced to them during their altered state of consciousness. For example, tribal societies present cultural dramas to orient their adolescents as they transition into adult hood. This phenomenon in which participants are guided in the experience and use of hallucinogens has been termed "managed altered states of consciousness." It is in such a state the tribal elders will inculcate their youth with culture, values, and societal norms through the psychedelic experience which is in stark contrast to the Western inter generational clash of the 1960s in which teenagers rebelled against parents. In shamanistic redemption, the parents assist in guiding their children through altered states and they grow together. So tribal life is introduced with a faced paced, profoundly educational psychedelic experience which teaches doctrines and morals while generating a strong personal identity.

However, redemption does not need to be considered in this spiritual context. Clients can be taught their own narratives of redemption while in clinical supervision. In other words, previous to entering an altered state of consciousness under clinical supervision, clients will have prepared or their families will have provides a narrative to be presented to the client by the clinicians during their managed altered state of consciousness. So the client's psychedelic learning experience is a story of redemption that is culturally, spiritually, and socially tailored to their life. It may be secular or religious, but the essence of redemption is that the process frees the client from a drug with undesirable states and restores them to desirable states. One of the primary reasons why these hallucinogens are such an effective learning experience is based on the event of "absolute unity of being" during which all perception of multiplicity of being is eradicated. Reality is perceived directly as one. This is accompanied by a profound and intrinsic sense of underlying unity, beauty, and goodness. *The person is enveloped in a complete sense of unity and well-being, which is perceived as oneness with the entire universe, union with God, or nirvana.* It is the context beyond all contexts. Neurophysiological research may find that the brain has the capacity to suspend the sense of diversity in reality in place of a holistic reality, neither one being more legitimate. However, it may be that traditional cultures have been successful in identifying activities which isolate these functions of the brain possibly in the parieto-occipital region. This powerful experience de facto binds us all together in a harmonious group in which all are satisfied and the universe is essentially good.

Conclusion

Perhaps, the best conclusion to such a potential treatment intervention is, why not? Why not consult with tribal shamans(Pajes) on treatments that have millennia of supervised success in a social context? Why not consider generating experiences in a managed setting which humans are determined to have? Why not explore natural interventions which mitigate all withdrawal symptoms and cravings thereby eliminating relapse? Is that too farfetched? Is it too impossible? Or is it just too disappointing and embittering that the lesser evolved, unscientific, uneducated, and poor shamans thought of it first? They knew it all along and yet they were satisfied not to trade places with us, knowledge is power, my point here is fight laziness and wake up before is too late.

CHAPTER 3

The Holy Jababa

The powerful and sublime Jababa... Jababa the ultimate comprehension.

What is Jababa?

In the Pariana region of the Brazilian Amazon jungle, the Pajes (Shaman) formerly prepared a mix of plants (herbs, fungi, etc.). Known only among the initiated as Jababa (indigenous name; without specific translation to English language, the closest one is an adult female, distinctly feminine in nature). Probably nothing has had a more fantastic story than Jababa among those Indian tribes. Most of them to this day speak only tribal dialects, so to gather knowledge from them is a difficult task. Goithyja spent months with the help of translators to not only have had the opportunity to experience Jababa but also provide to others the same ritual. It is known as a magical mix, and its content is only known by the Paje. Paje is the healer and the highest authority among Indians concerning plants of power, herbs, and wisdom (holy man). Jababa has aroused immense respect ever known among Indians. Jababa commanded the fear and respect of many tribal Indians of the Brazilian Amazon jungle, used only in ritual healing ceremonies by the direct guidance of a paje (this mix of entheogens cannot be sold, is only used by direct guidance of a knowledgeable shaman (Paje). Without proper preparation of mind, body, and soul, the neophyte can end up in trouble. Prior to the ritual, the psychonaut must pass throughout a healing process. In reality, a depuration of the mind, body, and soul, and must have a right mind-set; the last one is imperative to a successful holy experience (trip). It is also used in special occasions to divination as a magical and therapeutic formula to heal the soul. The paje says once the soul is healed, the human individual gets on the right track. Consequently, getting to know his/her true mission as human beings involving his/her consciousness within "paraatman."

How we do differentiate a so-called mystical experience, the voice from inside (paraatman, supreme soul, God), from just listening from our *subconscious mind* especially when most of us lack the saucam (purity), specifically mental purity. We must be open to a transcendental substance's existence with clean minds.

Jababa has the most significant power ever seen in transforming permanently one's personality, for better; but as all good things, it is not meant for everyone.

To experience Jababa, you shall be mentally healthy and does not present any serious illness. Jababa does not evocate nauseated states as *ayahuasca tea* does; it is easy in your digestive system once you follow up in strict details the paje's recommendations to a complete body, mind, and soul cleanser previous to the holy experience. The right environment is also the key to have a nice experience with it. In reality, most experienced people do prefer Jababa than ayahuasca tea, Jababa is far stronger and easy in your digestive system, speeding up awareness.

In this level of consciousness, sense data can be confirmed by an observer without necessarily implying understanding as more pure consciousness.

Use among Indians

Used to promote soul healing, cure diseases (most of our diseases are correlated with what we feed our body, mind, and souls), and mostly to promote interpersonal and extremely deep journeys into higher levels of consciousness to feel and experience God within; sometimes to talk to ancestors and the departed, near-death experiences, to travel into faraway distances, out-of-the-body experiences, and finally as a seed of wisdom. Not only Indians but also people who have had the divine grace to experience Jababa believe they see and talk to God. Jababa is revered as holy mix of entheogens among Indians and other peoples who have had the opportunity to communicate with the holy Jababa. As stated above, Jababa is not to everyone; you must be brave to embrace the holy experience.

Jababa Is . . .

No studies, not even pharmacologic have been performed on Jababa. All we know comes from paje's knowledge. Why does it still sound very secretive to these days to experience Jababa? After arduous, laborious effort to convince paje (Juruna), Goithyja finally got the green light to bring to regular people the holy experience with the powerful Jababa. The same must be done by the direct guidance of Goithyja or a person trained by him or a knowledgeable paje, only then the sacrament can be taken to the people from the cities. The sacrament must be shared in couple steps *in approved sites* surrounded by trees and away from the tumultuous big cities in the vicinities but not very close to the city (so, it does not need to be in the middle of Amazon jungle). the Paje acknowledges that all suffering is related to the lack of direct contact with God. Our civilization is much more older then we think it is—thousands of years older; once we do manage to establish contact with God within, we start the true soul's healing process. Our suffering is related also to our incapacity to unfold the full potential and the divine glory within oneself. The first step is getting to know who we really are.

The powerful holy Jababa is about unleashing the igneous power (in human beings, Shakti, the feminine aspect called Kundalini). This potential energy is said to rest at the base of the spinal cord. The object of the Tantric practice of Kundalini is to awaken this cosmic energy and make it ascend through the psychic centers, or the chakras, that lie along the axis of the spine as consciousness potentials. She will then unite above the crown of the head with Shiva the pure consciousness. This union is the aim of Kundalini, a resolution of duality into *unity again*, a fusion with the "absolute." By this union, the adept attains liberation while living, which is considered in Indian life to be the highest experience: a union of the individual with the universe. Later on, I understood how useful Tantra can be in this whole process of spiritual purification; how it has everything to do with the Vedic soma (ninth mandala, Rig-Vedas). Soma is more than entheogen; when you get the experience you will see and taste what soma really is.

Lord Krishna is the infinite ocean of pleasure and bliss (a state of profound satisfaction, happiness, and joy, a constant state of mind, undisturbed by gain or loss) saucam.

According to Gaudiya Vaishnava philosophy, *consciousness* is not a product of matter but is instead *a symptom of the soul.* All living beings, jivas, are distinct from their current body, the nature of the soul being eternal, immutable, and indestructible without any particular beginning or end. Souls, which are captivated by the illusory nature of the world, or *maya,* are repeatedly reborn among the various species of life on this planet and *on other worlds* in accordance to the laws of karma and individual desire. This is consistent with the concept of *samsara* found throughout Hindu belief.

Release from the process of *samsara* (known as *moksha*) is believed to be achievable through a variety of yoga and meditation processes. However, within Gaudiya Vaishnavism, it is *bhakti* in its purest state (or pure love of God) which is given as the ultimate aim, rather than liberation from the cycle of rebirth. There are many lines of yoga, but all are integral part of the Vedas. *Hatha yoga—ha* and *tha*, the sun and moon—refer to the two opposite currents that regulate all processes in our body. *Raja yoga* means royal and is sometimes called the crown of hatha yoga. Raja adds concentration after body and mind are cleaned and trained to stay calm and attentive. *Bhakti yoga* (union through devotion and love*)* is the yoga of selfless love, compassion, humility, purity, and the desire and serious intention to merge with God. *Jnana yoga* (the yoga of knowledge*)* is practical philosophy/metaphysics. It is both theory and practice. Jnana yoga uses the intellect as a tool to understand that our true self is behind and beyond our mind. *Kriya yoga* refers to actions designed to rid the body and mind of obstructions. *Kriya yoga* is a complete system including mantras, meditation, and other techniques toward controlling the life-force and bringing calmness and control over body and mind. The goal is to unite with pure awareness (God). Since pure awareness is our original condition, it is also referred to as self-awareness. Karma is the total sum of all our actions (mental and physical) in this life and before. *Karma yoga* is the yoga of service or self-transcending action, whereby the yogi directs all actions toward God. By serving God and humanity (without selfishness, egoism, and attachment) the heart becomes pure, the ego fades, and, over time, or even over many lifetimes, one becomes increasingly in tune and unified with God. Enlightenment (Samadhi, nirvana, union with God) is naturally realized through karma yoga. Kriya yoga has a lot to do with our work, using entheogens like ayahuasca tea, oo-koo-he balls, Jababa, magic mushrooms, etc. An entheogen (God inside us, in, within, God, divine, creates, generates), in the strict sense, is a psychoactive substance used in a shamanic or spiritual context.

Gaudiya Vaishnavas believe that God has many forms and names, but that the name "Krishna" is the fullest description because it means *"he who is all-attractive,"* covering all of God's aspects, such as being all powerful, supremely merciful, and all-loving. God is worshiped as the eternal, all-knowing, omnipresent, all-powerful, and all-attractive Supreme Person. Names of God from other religious traditions, such as Allah and Jehovah, are also accepted as bona fide titles of the same Supreme Person.

One of the defining aspects of Gaudiya Vaishnavism is that Krishna is worshiped specifically as the source of all Avataric incarnations of God. This is based on quotations from the Bhagavata Purana such as *"krsnas tu bhagavan svayam,"* translated as "Krishna is the original personality of Godhead" and from the Bhagavad Gita where Arjuna, when speaking to Krishna, states,

"You are the supreme personality of Godhead, the ultimate abode, the purest, the Absolute Truth. You are the eternal, transcendental, original person, the unborn, the greatest. All the great sages such as Narada, Asita, Devala and Vyasa confirm this truth about you, and now you yourself are declaring it to me."

Krishna is described elsewhere as the "seed-giving father of all living beings" and is worshiped within the Gaudiya tradition literally, as such Krishna being the "sustaining energy of the universe."

Maya is the opposite of enlightenment.

Maya, quoted as illusion, centered on the fact that we do not experience the environment itself but rather a projection of it, created by us (our egos, self). Mind, as an aspect of the soul in the sense of being both divine and immortal, links human thinking with the unchanging ordering principle of the cosmos itself. Maya is the principal deity that manifests, perpetuates, and governs the illusion and dream of duality in the phenomenal universe. For some mystics, this manifestation is illusion who does appears to be real, Each person, each physical object, from the perspective of eternity, is like a brief, disturbed drop of water from an unbounded ocean. The goal is to dissolve your ego and surrender to the infinite love of God; more precisely, to experience God, to see intuitively that the distinction between the self and the universe is a false dichotomy (any splitting of a whole into exactly two no overlapping parts). The distinction between consciousness and physical matter, between mind and body, is the result of an unenlightened living being. Understanding this reality with only your mind is one thing, experiencing is living this reality. It is like having someone who heard about the juice of one rare fruit of Amazon jungle but never have had the opportunity to really taste it and, on the other hand, a neophyte who really know the truth; the experience is living that reality in that level of consciousness. The goal of enlightenment.

I cannot talk about Jababa without mentioning the holy Vedas, because Jababa is the experience of the Vedas (science of the soul), Once you have the experience with Jababa, you will feel more creative, more intelligent, with improved memory, energized, feel more oneness (divine unity) with the holy soul of God (whom, in reality, we are all part of). You would go and know beyond this temporal unreal illusory touching, reality (difficult to describe in words).

So you would embrace and leave in one more subtle level of reality. Experiencing God and things who were there before but never ever touched with your heart (again I do repeat, it is impossible to put in words or describe it), getting a better understanding of our little and older brothers(more advanced humanoid like beings) who indeed both, share this planet with all of us. Of course, Jababa is a bundle of herbs, fungi, sometimes animal secretions (from frogs and other animals). The preparation of Jababa do not harm any animal whatsoever, rather it promotes awareness of all living beings (you will treat better our little brothers and be aware of our older ones). The neophyte must unveil the veil of maya to understand what I mean. The world which we all live in, pretty soon, is going to change dramatically for the better, but, in the course of that, we will be seeing sudden dramatic changes. But there is nothing to worry about, nobody lives forever in this realm of illusory reality. With Jababa, you will see with your own eyes, so you don't need to believe me you will see it. To see it is believe. So Jababa can create or, better saying, unleash somebody's reactions to the more sensitive people, but nothing a normal and healthy human being cannot handle; so relax. I did experience with Jababa numerous times, and I managed to survive. I'm no longer young, so it is not a big deal. Anyone can do it. If one man can do it, another can too. By the way, this is my philosophy: never say never. If you really want, you can do it. Being positive will help make things run smoothly more often. So experiencing with Jababa enables us to get into higher states of consciousness deeper. We do dive in that reality; higher we all go. It sounds like a metaphor, but it is true. I humbly leave my statement here: among all I have experienced, Jababa is the most powerful and divine bundle of entheogens which I ever experienced with. It is stronger than the famous fabled DMT rich brew called oo-koo-he mentioned by Terence Mckenna in his book. In reality, oo-koo-he is made with mushroom's ashes, toad secretions rich in 5-MeO-DMT (5 methoxydimethyltryptamine), also N, N-Di-methyltryptamine (DMT) among a couple of other herbs. By the way, I do believe what he put his hands on was not the true oo-koo-he; the real one is a very powerful occurring psychedelic compound and (the natives don't like gringos snooping around in their territory) must be taken only in the jungle or in a land far away from big cities surrounded by trees. If you take Jababa or the "true" oo-koo-he on a big city you can go crazy; It is very powerful. A couple of years ago when I was having ayahuasca tea at the Brazilian church I heard the case of one lady from France who took the tea for two consecutive years spacing it, off fifteen days in the Brazilian church, but suddenly she resolved came back to her beloved Paris (by the way a beautiful city but a big city) and I don't know how she did convince one member of the church to allow her to bring the tea to France, so she did it without the proper preparation and the wise guidance of an experienced paje (shaman). She ended up jumping from her apartment in Paris! This is a sad, but a true story. To do use a powerful entheogen, you, must have guidance. You see, without the proper ritual and consecration you can end up in trouble. Furthermore, I will explain in details how to prepare yourself and bring into the right environment, to experience with more manageable plants of light as you wish and when you want it, just by following a couple of directions; to be sure you can have a pleasurable, nice and smoothly experience. Remember, knowledge is power!

Why talk about the Vedas? Because the experience with entheogen has no meaning without a spiritual context. We must guide the experience to the right target from the beginning to the end to avoid being lost or trapped inside our own polluted minds (influenced and fed by TV, news, radio, stressful daily lives, etc.) releasing visual stress, which are not good to the whole context of the work. When we take entheogen we must seek higher levels of consciousness and not get caught or trapped in our polluted realm. As explained before, we are influenced by the environment and our minds. Why some folks report having bad trips because they do not prepare themselves prior to taking entheogens.

Jababa is a mix of plants and herbs and only prepared by selected Indians. This sacred knowledge is called sacramental and is only passed on from paje to paje (shaman) at the time of paje's death or in some occasion, in particular, when the paje is close to his/her departed he/she will designate the new guardian of the Jababa's knowledge. It is not only the formula who does contain many herbs but the right manipulation of the ritual that combines nature's knowledge and spirituality. By the way, Paje Juruna does not want to end up like Maria Sabina, when she did release the secrets of velada and salvia to the white-man civilization. So Goithyja explained to Paje Juruna what happened with Maria Sabina after the release of such information, allowing Westerners to participate in the healing vigil that became known as the velada, where all participants partake of the psylocibin mushroom as a sacrament to open the gates of the mind. While she was initially hospitable to the truth seekers thronging to her, their lack of respect for the sacred and traditional purposes caused María Sabina to remark. Late in life, María Sabina became bitter about her many misfortunes and how others had profited from her name. Nevertheless, late in her life, she confided to Joan Halifax that the dissemination of the knowledge of the sacred mushroom was her fate, that it was preordained by God that she met Wasson. She also felt that the ceremony of the velada had been desecrated and irremediably polluted by the hedonistic use of the mushrooms.

"From the moment the foreigners arrived, the 'holy children' lost their purity. They lost their force, they ruined them. Henceforth they will no longer work. There is no remedy for it."

Goithyja does prefer keep a positive attitude toward entheogen; he does know that with proper preparation and mind set, the holy experience can be granted to every serious dweller of planet earth.

Maria Sabina had visions on the "little saints" that someone (Wasson) was coming and would take the tradition to the world after five hundred years of secrecy under Spanish rule. As a result of that action, giving the secrets of the "little saints" to outsiders, her son was murdered and her house burned to the ground. During the later years of her life, she lamented that "the power of the sacrament had been lost in the clouds" and ended up speaking English instead of the Mazatec. She lived to age ninety-one, passing away on November 22, 1985.

So Paje Juruna does not want to end up like that. By the way, Juruna is a pseudonym. I would rather not reveal his name to avoid troubles to that dear holy man.

OUR GRATITUDE TO THIS KNOWLEDGE
We do want you to know that most!

God desires to be expressed in the world through us. The example set by Lord Jesus is apparently a "pattern" of wholeness for each and every soul, regardless of an individual's religious or personal beliefs.

This Christ pattern was further described as "the awareness within each soul, imprinted in pattern on the mind and waiting to be awakened by the will of the soul's oneness with God." Why Jababa? Because it is a powerful entheogen which does not promote nauseated states and is easy to control. Mushrooms can be handy and powerful but difficult to control; Jababa can be taken in steps until the individual reach the right dose. Some scholars say soma is the essence of the Vedas, which has everything to do with entheogenic substances and sexual energy "libido." Jababa, (n) an adult female, is distinctly feminine in nature. Dakini is the feminine power of the soul, described as a female embodiment of enlightened energy. The feminine enhanced by the use of entheogenic substances is the key to reach such goal: God within.

CHAPTER 4

The Opening of the Third Eye
Practical Exercise Eyes of Horus

Since Horus was said to be the sky, he was considered to also contain the sun and moon. It became said that the sun was his right eye and the moon his left and that they traversed the sky when he, a falcon, flew across it.

The best exercise to reach that degree of mental acuity is *tratak*. The technique of tratak does remain much the same, whatever the target of you gaze is, though naturally you will have to adapt it slightly.

First exercise: Once you are completely relaxed, concentrate on the area between your eyes on your forehead. This is also called the "third eye." It has been linked with psychic abilities throughout the ages. In actuality, there is a gland in that approximate area of the head called the pineal gland, which has been believed to be the link between the physical and spiritual being. Still concentrating on this area, roll your still closed eyes upward to this position. Do not strain them, it should not be uncomfortable. Only roll them as far back as is comfortable. While in this position and still completely relaxed, try to enhance the state of dream, awake and being conscious at once, this does only came with practice.

Practice brings perfection. Remember you must have such control to experience the higher states of consciousness. Focus is the key.

Second exercise: Gazing the object indoors, place the object one foot higher than the eyesight level, five feet away from you. Seat comfortably, first of all. Regulate your breathing, breathe passively and then start to gaze at the object without blinking. Better make this exercise with empty digestive system. Don't stare or gaze vacantly, just look steady without straining; after about ten minutes, close your eyes and keep your inner gaze steady. Visualize the object; when the after image disappear, open your eyes and repeat the exercise again. The object can be a crystal ball, small one, or a point on the wall. Try to reach twenty minutes on a daily basis.

Third exercise: When meditating outdoors, try to gaze at the sun. Start with one minute going until three minutes on a daily basis, better in the early hours of the day. The sun-gazing is the most widely used object of tratak in all times. It is used by the Mayans, Aztecs, Egyptians, and many natives of South America, among others. It is easy to hold one afterimage of the sun when you close your eyes.

If you notice any abnormality with your eyesight, stop immediately, trading for wall gazing, practice brings perfection. Remember, mental acuity is the key in any meditation practices.

CHAPTER 5

The Dropping Soma

Soma: In Indian mythology, at the beginning of time, the gods got together and churned the ocean to extract a substance, which would confer immortality. The gods agreed to share this mighty elixir, but one of them apparently absconded with the whole pot of holy Ambrosia. Fleeing with the "nectar of the gods," over the course of twelve days, the decoction Amrita was spilt onto four auspicious places, namely, Prayag, Hardwar, Ujjain, and Nasik. The most popular version of the Indian myth, churning the milk ocean is found in the eighth canto of the Bhagavata Purana. In Buddhist mythology, Amrita is the drink of the gods, which grants them immortality. The ninth mandala of the Rig Veda is known as the soma mandala. According to Terrence McKenna, in his book *The Food of Gods*, the psilocybin containing Stropharia cubensis (Psilocybe cubensis) mushroom is a likely Soma candidate. Remember, soma is not only an entheogen. It is more than that. Soma is a mix between igneous power Prana and entheogens. Psilocybin, the active psychoactive component in Stropharia (Psylocibe) Cubensis has a strong hallucinogenic nature. Soma (Sanskrit) or Haoma (Avestan) was a ritual drink of importance among the early Indo Iranians and the later Vedic and Iranian cultures. It is frequently mentioned in the Rig Veda, which contains many hymns praising its energizing or intoxicating qualities. The use of substances in ritual or religious observances is a practice that is abundantly attested in the shamanic world as well as among some yogis, and among the rishis in the Vedas. We know that Patanjali himself puts simples (ausadhi) together with Samadhi, among the means of obtaining the siddhis. The Aryan Ur religion, in the Rig Veda the sacramental basis of the Vedic religion (better saying science of the soul) was the preparation and consumption of a decoction obtained by mixing the juice of the fly agaric with other ingredients, one of which may have been hemp, or even *wine* like the Eleusis mysteries and Parcephone's quest to enlightenment, or a beverage prepared by extracting the juice from the Amanita Muscaria fungus, bundle with other herbs. This Ur religion does not begin with the composition of the Vedas, when the Aryans arrived in India, but much further back in time, in the late Ice Age in Siberia. During this cold age, when people had to live most of the time deep inside caves or other dwellings, an inward direction was given to their spiritual endeavors. Due to this fact and with the aid of certain magical herbs and plants, man first invented religion. When the Aryans came down from Siberia they brought with them their Ur religion and an Urgaritic language, which became the Vedic and Persian religious expression and later the Indo-European language, which includes Sanskrit and Persian, and the dialects of Greek, Finnish, German, Hindi, and Urdu. Soma Rasa, Nectar of the Gods Soma in the case of the Vedas, and Haoma in the case of the Iranians—that is, the Persians. These Aryans, a word which originally meant "noble tiller of the earth," an agriculturist, "digging stick in hand," came from Siberia, not by invasion, and not in 1500 BCE, but by a process of diffusion, as described by the famous archaeologist Colin Renfrew, around 7000 BCE. The first Aryans settled in what is called the Saraswati

Valley. According to Gordon Wasson, "There is little doubt that the substance called soma in the Rig Veda has been identified as the fungus Amanita Muscaria." (Soma is more than that.) However, there is evidence that successive waves of Aryan immigrants came to India in later years, perhaps up to as recently as 2000 BCE. (Our civilization is thousands and thousands of years older than scholars think it is.) The evidence for this is centered on three incontrovertible facts:

There is a direct affinity between Sanskrit and Finnish. The Aryan speakers who composed the Vedas were akin to the same Aryan speakers who moved to what is now Iran, the latter having composed the Avesta, both of which scriptures center on the cult of the magical substance, soma. According to Wendy Doniger O'Flaherty, a Rig Vedic scholar, "The soma sacrifice was the focal point of the Vedic religion."

The Amanita Muscaria has been traced by mycologists to Siberia. This has been proved by not only Wasson but also other eminent botanists, such as S. Hajicek Dobberstein, the author of the paper "Soma Siddhas and Alchemical Enlightenment: Psychedelic Mushrooms in Buddhist Tradition," published in the *Journal of Ethno Pharmacology*. The Amanita Muscaria spoken of in the Rig Veda has its origin in the northern area around Finland and Siberia, where the fungus still grows and can be seen each year.

There is no evidence that the Amanita Muscaria grows in the Himalayas or in the desert that comprised the Land of the Five Rivers—that is, Arya Bharata. Based on these facts, it is clear that the Aryans came from outside India, brought with them a language very similar to Finnish, a people who had an intimate knowledge of the "fly agaric" growing in Siberia, but not in India, and composed the

Vedas while under the influence of a psychedelic substance when they arrived in modern Pakistan, after parting company with their Persian cousins, who stayed in Iran. From these people, we got our language, which spread over the Middle East, India, and Europe. And from these people, we got the Vedic religion, a religion that centered on the soma and sacramental use of entheogens. As further evidence, please note that the Tibetan word for "cannabis" is "So.Ma.Ra.Dza"–that is, somaraja, king of soma, and "bDud.rTsi," which in Tibetan means "drink juice." It is used for sacramental use, with sages eating cannabis flowers and resin (hashish), not smoking it. The smoking of cannabis was introduced to the Western civilization later on by the Turks and translated from the Sanskrit and taken to Tibet by the eighty-four Mahasiddhas of Vajrayana Buddhism in the tenth century of our era. The mysterious substance referred to in Buddhist texts, variously described as amrita, is none other than a similar decoction containing a similar alkaloid as contained in the soma fungus. Apparently, the proper performance of sacrificial ritual was of the utmost importance in the Vedic Aryan religion. By means of the sacrifice, it was believed that certain individuals could win the favor of the gods. Even before the Aryans entered India, the sacrifice had become a complex and elaborate affair. The sacrifice involved the slaughter of dozens and sometimes hundreds of animals: cattle, sheep, goats, and horses. At that time, the initial knowledge of soma was corrupted by maya, mental illusions created by our egos and minds; why, sooner after that, mankind lost sight with the true identity of soma rasa only regaining again after millennia. With the help of Goithyja and many others like him, most of Western ethnobotanists believe soma is just a fungi or herb, but they are missing the most important content of all, the igneous power (viril and prana), as priests uttered the sacred formulae and the mysterious chants of the Vedic hymns. According to historians, J. Bently and H. Ziegler, worshippers partook of soma, a sort of elixir of the gods, a hallucinogenic decoction that produced a divine sense of power and inspiration (bring us closer to God, weakening our powerful egos). Our egos separate humankind from God within. The hymns are recorded in the Rig Veda, particularly in mandala IX and X, wherein it is described as a sacred event as the gods themselves joined the participants and partook in the ritual eating and drinking.

By pleasing the gods with sacrifice, song, drink, and food (both coarse and soft), the Vedic Aryans hoped to gain the support of nature (and much military success), large families, long life, and abundant herds of cattle. These sacrifices required the constant attention of a special class of priests who were required to perform no less than five rituals per day for the average common household. The most purified rituals which happened thousands of years ago have had no killings whatsoever of animals or humans. That was a later misleading interpretation of that knowledge, like what happened with the Mayans, those who built the pyramids, they did not make human or animal sacrifice. It was only later on when man lost contact with God that the widespread killings started. What we do learn today is not what really used to happen. The idea that Soma was an entheogen, specifically the red-capped Amanita Muscaria mushroom, as described in mandalas IX and X of Rig Veda, was first presented by the ethnomycologist R. Gordon Wasson. The Amanita grows in a mycorrhizal relationship with a number of different trees, specifically the pines, firs, and above all, the birches, from which the mushroom must feed from. An example of the readings (from the ninth mandala of Rig Veda): Flow soma, in a most sweet and exhilarating stream, effused for Indra to drink. The destroyer of Rakshasas has stepped upon his gold-smitten birthplace, united with the wooden cask. Be the lavish giver of wealth, most bounteous, the destroyer of enemies; bestow on us the riches of the affluent. Come with food to the sacrifice of the mighty gods, and bring us strength and sustenance. To thee we come, O dropping (soma); for thee only is this our worship day by day, our prayers are to thee, none other. Amanita: an alkaloid, of the mushroom species. Its common name is "fly agaric," and it has been described by mycologists such as Pileus as

> Size : 5 X 7, 25 X 40 cm broad
> Shape: convex, becoming plane to slightly wavy or depressed in age
> Color : blood red, or various shades of bright, scarlet, or orange red; becoming lighter toward margin
> Surface: smooth, covered with white warts or small patches (remains of the universal veil); sometimes washing off in age; tacky, sticky or viscid when moist
> Margin: striate; at first appendiculate
> Flesh : firm when young and becoming soft in age, white (yellowish beneath cuticle), thick;
> Odor : faint
> Taste : pleasant

Alkaloids and Maharish Patanjali. Mircea Eliade states in his classic book *Yoga: Immortality or Freedom* that in the sphere of shamanism, strictly speaking, "intoxication by the use of entheogens [like: hemp, mushrooms, tobacco, fungi, hoasca tea, salvia, baby wood rose, kava kava, epadu, Jababa [a bundle of herbs and fungi used by the most knowledgeable pajes in the Brazilian Amazon rain forest), Oo-koo-he, *Ephedra*, mescalin, etc.] So, the true effects presented by the use of entheogens seem to have formed part of the original practice.(what really matters is the soma effect, does not matter which entheogen was used, of course some entheogen are more suitable than others!) For on the one hand, shamanic myths and folklore record a decadence among the shamans of the present-day (but not all) who have become unable to obtain ecstasy in the fashion of the "great shamans of long ago." (What about of the widespread killing of shamans perpetrated by the Christian church, crusades, inquisition?) On the other, it has been observed that where shamanism is in decomposition and the trance is simulated, there is also overindulgence in intoxicants and drugs. (The key to succeed is having the right mind-set and the proper preparation of the ritual). Mircea Eliade wrote that only the rudiments of classic Yoga are to be found in the Vedas, and while Shamanism and other techniques of ecstasy are documented among other Indo-European people, Yoga is to be found only in India and in cultures influenced by Indian spirituality. Eliade notes, "Possession by spirits, although documented in a great man, shamanism does not seem to have been a primary and essential element. Rather, it suggests a phenomenon of degeneration; as mentioned before, for the supreme goal of the shaman is to abandon his body and rise to heaven or descend into hell (hell, another fabrication of the Christian church, is only in the mind of the laggards; those who experience God within sees only the wonders of the creator of the universe and everything good in it), not to let himself be 'possessed' by his assisting spirits, by demons or the souls of the dead (low levels of consciousness in the low-vibrational realms of existence), having Lord Krishna and sage Jesus in our hearts and minds, we will only experience the greatness of God; the shaman's ideal is to master these spirits, not to let himself be 'occupied' by them."

Psychic and spiritual powers (siddhi) may be inborn, or they may be gained by the use of simples, or by mantra, or by striving, or by meditation. "Simples" mean ecstasy-inducing herbs (by the use of entheogen) from which the elixir of longevity was extracted. Mircea Eliade believes that these "mystical means" properly belong to the phenomenology of ecstasy and they were only reluctantly admitted into the sphere of classic yoga. According to Eliade, "Yet the fact that Patanjali himself refers to the magico ecstatic virtues of simples is both significant and pregnant with consequences; it proves the pressure exercised by the ecstatic, their will to substitute their methods for the disciplines of classic yoga." The use of sacramental substances in ritual or religious observances is a practice that is abundantly attested in the shamanic world as well as among some Indian religions such as the Avesta and the Vedas In the Rig Veda, the sacramental basis of the Vedic religion was the preparation and consumption of a decoction obtained by mixing the juice of the various plants with other ingredients.

CHAPTER 6

Maintaining SPIRITUAL FOCUS

Why talk about Vedas? To guide any serious neophyte to the highest spiritual realm, we must at least have some knowledge about the creator of the universe and the only trustful religious work which explains in details that field of knowledge, which is the science of the soul, "Vedas." If you go only after the most famous religious books out there, most of the time you only find historical reference of content, not any practical teaching to achieve the higher levels of consciousness. If you seek more refined knowledge you must go after the Vedas, only then we can dive into soma states by the help of the right bundle of entheogenic substances and have also the guidance of a truly knowledgeable mystic or shaman (guru), to avoid toe kicks in pursuing the entheogenic path, best if we can combine both in one."

Now a brief introduction of the Vedas, the science of the soul.

Vyasa categorized the primordial single Vedas into four. Hence he was called Veda Vyasa. Veda Vyasa cognized the Vedas from Lord Krishna. So to the best of my knowledge, which is a public knowledge, mostly what we do see today are translations from Sanskrit into other languages done by scholars. So if we can call it that, the author of the Vedas is Lord Krishna. Every particle of the universe(s) is him, manifested and unmanifested!

If we are going to understand the essential truths in Vedic literature, then we must get a glimpse of the content and purpose of its many texts and the expansive nature of the knowledge it contains. The Vedic philosophy encompasses the oldest spiritual texts of any religion in the world, and its subjects are broad and numerous. Its more advanced concepts can be difficult for even the greatest scholars to fathom. The Vedic literature discusses many types of philosophical viewpoints, and studying some of them will let us see that many of the concepts that we accept as new today are nothing more than parts of the ancient Vedic knowledge that had been dealt with and thoroughly understood thousands of years ago. Thus, there are not many ideas that are really new at all. The main purpose of the Vedic literature is to establish knowledge of the Absolute Truth and the process for attaining the highest levels of self realization. To do that, it must, and does, contain the elementary as well as most advanced forms of spiritual knowledge. So let us see exactly what kind of information is found within the many volumes of Vedic literature, and if there is any one understanding or direction in particular which it encourages people to take for complete spiritual success. If you are new to the study of Vedic culture, you may not understand all of these ancient Vedic texts or their purpose, or why it is necessary to mention them in this book. However, this study will provide the knowledge for you to begin to see how vast the Vedic science is and how numerous are these Vedic texts. You will begin to understand that there are few topics that have been left uncovered in the Vedic investigation of reality and the search for truth and in its presentation of what is God. You will also understand in the final analysis what direction they most recommend and how to pursue it.

The Vedic literature is composed of many books. The oldest, the *Rig-Veda, Yajurveda, Samaveda,* and the *Atharvaveda.* It is said in the *Muktikopanishad* that these four *Vedas* had 21, 109, 1,000, and 50 branches respectively, with over 100,000 verses. Now, however, we can only find around 20,023 (some say 20,379) verses in total from these four *Vedas.* The *Rig-Veda,* the Veda of praise, contains 1,017 hymns, or 10,522 verses, arranged in ten books or *mandalas.* The first eight mostly contain hymns of praise to the various demigods, such as Indra and Agni. The ninth book deals primarily with the soma ritual, which was the extraction and purification of the juice of the soma herb. The tenth book contains *suktas,* or verses, of wisdom and mantras that would cause certain magical effects to take place. The *Rig-Veda* hymns were mainly of praise to the gods that were invoked during the Vedic ceremonies for ensuring immediate material needs. These were chanted by the four priests who conducted the Vedic rituals, namely the *hota,* who calls the gods with the mantras from the *Rig-Veda*; the *adhvaryu,* who performs all the rituals of the ceremony according to the *Yajurveda*; the *udgata,* who sings the *Samaveda* mantras; and the *Brahmana,* who supervises the general ceremony. However, it was usually only the Brahmana priests who could be sure of chanting the mantras accurately to produce the desired result. If the mantra was chanted incorrectly by someone who was not qualified, the desired result would not take place and often something undesirable or horrible would happen instead. The main gods in the *Rig-Veda* were Indra (the god of heaven and rain); Agni (the fire god); and Surya (the sun god). Surya is invoked in the sacred Gayatri mantra. However, Surya is also called Surya Narayana in the *Rig-Veda.* So the hymns to Surya and his different forms can also be related to Narayana or Vishnu, especially those to *Savitur*. Vishnu is also known as the Pervader, meaning that all the Vedic gods are absorbed in him, and thus must also emanate from him. They would be absorbed in him during the time of cosmic annihilation, but would also emanate from him during the time of the creation. There were also verses to three other names and forms of the sun god, namely, Savitri, Mitra, and Pooshan. Other gods included Dyos (a celestial god), Varuna (god of the seas), Soma, Marut (god of air or wind called Vayu in other places), Ru-dra (a form of Shiva) and Vishnu as supreme God. All of these gods are celestial gods, or demigods, except for Rudra and Vishnu. There is also the important Purusha Sukta hymn in the ninetieth chapter of the *Rig-Veda's* tenth *mandala*. The *Rig-Veda* is also a mystical text that contains knowledge in its abstract imagery of what the seers had realized. It has information on yoga, the spinal current and the chakras, as well as the planets and their orbits. Many aspects of this mystical knowledge are also contained in the other *Vedas*. The *Rig-Veda* is said to have had twenty-one branches, out of which only two are still available. Much of the *Shakal* branch is still available, along with the *Brahmana* and *Aranyaka* of the *Shankhayan* branch. Although there are some stories in the *Rig-Veda*, there are few historical records of the early Vedic kings. This has been a mistake among various linguists and researchers who study the *Rig-Veda* to try to get a historical understanding of the early Vedic kingdom and Aryans.

The *Yajurveda* is the Veda of rituals and contains 1,975 verse mantras in forty chapters, many of which are similar to those in the *Rig-Veda* and used in rituals, usually by the *adhvaryu* priest. These contain different levels of knowledge and wisdom. The Yajurveda once had 109 branches of knowledge, but now only parts of seven branches are found, of which the *Vajasaneyi* is prominent. The *Yajurveda*, however, has two *samhitas*, or collections of verses, known as the *White Yajurveda* (or *Vajasaneyisamhita*) with the hymns and rituals, and the *Black Yajurveda* (or *Taittiriyasamhita*) with their interpretations. These were primarily for the priests to use as a guide in performing sacred rituals, such as the *ashvamedha* or *rajasuya*, since they also contain directions or formulas that the priests use along with the verses that are sung during the ceremony.

The *Samaveda*, the Veda of melodies, contains 1,549 verses meant to be used as songs in various ceremonies, primarily for the *udgata* priest. Most of them are taken from the *Rig-Veda* and arranged according to their use as utilized in particular rituals. From the original one thousand branches of the *Samaveda*, three are still available, of which the *Kauthumiya* and *Jaiminiya* are prominent.

The *Atharvaveda* is the Veda of chants and once had fifty branches of which we have only the *Shaunak* branch today. It is a book of 5,977 verses in twenty chapters containing prayers, spells, and incantations, which in some respects resemble magical instructions found in the Tantras and even various magical incantations. The *Atharvaveda* contains a small section of verses of instruction, wisdom, descriptions of the soul, and God, but the majority of it consists of rules for worshipping the planets, rules for oblations and sacrifices, prayers for averting evil and disease, incantations for the destruction of foes, for fulfilling personal desires, etc., mostly for the material needs of people. The four primary *Vedas* represent the accomplishment of a highly developed religious system and encourage satisfaction of material desires through worship of the demigods.

They contain many directions for increasing one's power and position, or for reaching the heavens in one's future by properly performing particular sacrifices in worship to the *devas* (demigods), and so on. Some people ask why there seems to be so many gods within Hinduism or Vedic culture. Yet if we properly analyze the situation, we will understand that there is but one Supreme Being who has many agents or demigods who assist in managing the creation and the natural forces within. And like anyone else, if they are properly approached with prayer or worship, they may help facilitate the person by granting certain wishes that may be within the jurisdiction of that demigod. In some places in the Vedic literature, it is explained that there are thirty-three Vedic gods, or even as many as thirty-three million. The thirty-three gods are calculated as being eight Vasus, eleven Rudras (forms of Shiva), twelve Adityas, along with Indra and Prajapati (Brahma). Then there are also other positions that are considered major or minor *devas*. According to the *Vedas*, the *devas* are not imaginary or mythological beings but are agents of the Supreme Will to administer different aspects of the universal affairs. They do represent and control various powers of nature. Thus, they manifest in the physical, subtle, or psychic levels of our existence both from within and without. In this way, a transcendentalist sees that behind every aspect of nature is a personality. The names of these gods are considered offices or positions rather than the actual name of the demigod. For example, we may call the president of the country by his personal name, or simply Mr. President. It's the position itself that allows for him to have certain powers or areas of influence. In the case of the *devas*, it is only after accumulating much pious credit that a living being can earn the position of being a particular demigod. Then a person may become an Indra, or Vayu, or attain some other position to assume specific powers, or to control various aspects of material energy. Another example is that when you walk into a big factory, you see so many workers and all that they are doing. You may initially think that these workers are the reason for whatever goes on in the factory. However, more important than the workers are the foremen, the managers, and then the executives. Among these you will find people of varying degrees of authority. Someone will be in charge of designing the products. Another may be the chief financial officer or main accountant. Another may be in charge of personnel, while someone else may be in charge of maintenance in the factory itself. Finally, a chief executive officer or president of the company is the most important of all. Without him, there may not even be a company. You may not see the president right away, but his influence is everywhere since all the workers are engaging in projects according to his decisions. The managers and foremen act as his authorized agents to keep things moving accordingly. The numerous demigods act in the same way concerning the functions of nature, all of whom represent some aspect or power of the Supreme Will. That's why it is sometimes said there are thirty-three million different gods in Hinduism. Actually, there may be many forms, *avataras*, or aspects of God, but there is only one God, or one Absolute Truth. This is often a confusing issue to people new to Vedic philosophy. We often hear the question among Westerners that if Hinduism has so many gods, how do you know which ones to worship? The point is that the *devas* affect all levels of universal activities, including the weather, or who is bestowed with particular opulence such as riches, beautiful wife or husband, large family, good health, etc. For example, one could worship Agni for getting power, Durgadevi for good fortune, Indra for good sex life or plenty of rain, or the Vasus for getting money. Such instruction is in the *karmakanda* section of the *Vedas,* which many people considered to be the most important part of Vedic knowledge. This is for helping people acquire the facilities for living a basic material existence. There are, of course, various actions, or *karmas,* prompted by our desires to achieve certain results, but this is not the complete understanding of the *karmakanda* section of the *Vedas.* The *karmakanda* section is meant to supply the rituals for purifying our mind and actions in the pursuit of our desires and not merely to live with the intent of acquiring all of one's material wants and necessities from the demigods. By having faith and steadiness in the performance of the ritual, one establishes purification in one's habits and thoughts. This provides a gradual process of acquiring one's needs and working out one's desires while simultaneously becoming purified and free of them. Such purification can then bring one to a higher level of spiritual activity. This was the higher purpose of the *karmakanda* rituals. Without this understanding, one misses the point and remains attached to rituals in the pursuit of material desires, which will drag one further into material existence. The reciprocation between the demigods and society is explained in Bhagavad Gita. It is stated that in the beginning the Lord of all beings created men and demigods along with the sacrifices to Lord Vishnu that were to be performed. The Lord blessed them saying that these sacrifices will enable men to prosper and attain all desirable things. By these sacrificial duties, the demigods will be pleased and the demigods will also please you with all the necessities of life, and prosperity will spread to all. But he who enjoys what is given by the demigods without offering them in return is a thief. In this way, it was recommended that people could perform sacrificial rituals to obtain their desires. However, by the performance of such acts, they should understand their dependent position, not only on the demigods, but ultimately on the Supreme Being. As further explained in *Bhagavad Gita,* all living beings exist on food grains, which are produced from rain, which is produced by the performance of prescribed sacrifices or duties. These prescribed duties are described in the Vedic literature, which is manifested from the Supreme Being. Therefore, the Supreme is eternally established in acts of sacrifice. Although the demigods may accept worship from the human beings and bless them with particular benedictions according to the sacrifices that are performed, they are still not on the level of the supreme lord Vishnu (who is an incarnation of Lord Krishna). The *Rig-Veda* explains, "The demigods are always looking to that supreme abode of Vishnu." *Bhagavad Gita* also points out: "From the beginning of creation, the three syllables *om tat sat* have been used to indicate the Supreme Absolute Truth (Brahman). They were uttered by *brahmanas* while chanting the Vedic hymns and during sacrifices, for the satisfaction of the Supreme." In this way, by uttering *om tat sat,* which is stressed in Vedic texts, the performers of the rituals for worshiping the demigods were also offering obeisance to Lord Vishnu for its success. The four *Vedas* mainly deal with material elevation, and since Lord Vishnu is the Lord of material liberation, most sacrifices were directed toward the demigods. In *Bhagavad Gita,* however, Lord Krishna points out that men of small knowledge, who are given to worldly desires, take delight in the flowery words of the *Vedas* that prescribe rituals for attaining power, riches, or rebirth in heaven. With their goal of enjoyment, they say there is nothing else than this. However, Krishna goes on to explain in *Bhagavad Gita* that when a person desires to worship a particular demigod for the temporary and limited fruits he or she may bestow, Krishna, as the supersoul in everyone's heart, makes that person's faith in that demigod steady. But all the benefits given by any demigod actually are given by Krishna alone, for without whom no one has any power. The worshipers of the demigods go to the planets of the demigods, but worshippers of Krishna reach Krishna's spiritual abode. Thus, as one progresses in understanding, it is expected that they will gradually give up the pursuit for temporary material pleasures and then begin to endeavor for reaching the supreme goal of Vedic knowledge. For one who is situated in such knowledge and is self-realized, the prescribed duties in the *Vedas* for worshiping the demigods are unnecessary. As *Bhagavad Gita* explains, for one who is fully self-realized, who is fully satiated in the self, delights only in the self, there is no duty or need to perform the prescribed duties found in the *Vedas*, because he has no purpose or material desires to fulfill. However, another view of the Vedic gods is that they represent different aspects of understanding ourselves, especially through the path of yoga and meditation. For example, the god of wind is Vayu, and is related to the practice of yoga as the breath and its control in *pranayama*. Agni is the god of fire and relates to the fire of consciousness or awareness. Soma relates to the bliss in the *samadhi* of yoga practice. Many of the Vedic gods also represent particular powers of yoga and are related to the different *chakras* in the subtle body. It is accepted that as a person raises his or her consciousness through the *chakras*, he or she will attain the level of awareness and the power and assistance that is associated with the particular divine personality related to that *chakra*. Although the four principal *Vedas* include the concept of spiritual perfection or liberation, it is not so thoroughly developed or presented. Therefore, to help one understand what the goal of Vedic philosophy is, there are also other compositions along with the four *Vedas*, namely the *Brahmanas, Aranyakas,* and the *Upanishads*. Originally, the *Brahmanas* consisted of 1,180 branches, with the same number of *Aranyakas.* Unfortunately, only a few of these branches remain today. The *Upanishads* also had 1,180 branches to continue the explanation of these Vedic divisions of knowledge and practice. However, only about two hundred are still available.

The *Brahmanas* are compositions that accompany different portions of the *Veda Samhitas* with additional directions and details that the *brahmana* priests would use when performing the sacrificial rituals, along with some of their histories. They include the *Aitareya*, the *Shankhayan* or *Kausitaki*, and the *Shatpath* and *Taittariya Brahmanas* that are connected to the *Rig-Veda*. These contain such instructions as what to meditate on and how to chant the mantras while conducting the sacrifice, etc. The *Brahmanas* also hold cosmological legends and stories that explain the reason for performing the Vedic rituals, along with the esoteric significance of the mantras and sacrificial rituals. They also describe the verses in the main *Samhitas*. Furthermore, they provide the seeds of the systematic knowledge of the *Sutras*, and can be used by the village householders. The *Panchvinsha, Shadvinsha,* and *Tandya Brahmanas* belong to the *Sama Veda*, while the *Jaiminiya* and *Gopatha Brahmanas* belong to the *Atharva Veda*. The *Shatapatha Brahmana*, a large volume of one hundred chapters authored by Yajnavalkya, is said to belong to the *Shukla Yajur Veda*. The *Aranyakas* are sacred writings that are supposed to frame the essence of the *Upanishads* and are considered to be secret and dangerous to the uninitiated. The *Aranyakas* reveal more of the esoteric aspects of the rituals and their purposes than the *Brahmanas*. They are meant only for the *brahmana* priests and *kshatriya* warriors who have renounced all materialistic activities, and retired to the solitude of the forests, which is the meaning of "*aranyaka*." They include a strict style of worship to particular forms or aspects of God. These instructions could consist of which mantras to use for particular purposes, how to sit, in which time of the morning to practice, the devotions to incorporate into the practice, and so on. Next we come to the *Upanishads*, which is the main part of the *Aranyakas* and constitute one of the most sacred portions of Vedic philosophy. There are three main sections of the Vedic scriptures. The *Upanishads* and *Arany-akas* are part of the *jnana kanda* section, meaning they contain knowledge meant for introspection and contemplation. The four main *Samhitas* and *Brahmanas*, which deal primarily with rituals are a part of the *karmakanda* classification, meant for appeasing the gods for one's necessities and desires, and for helping purify the mind. The *upasanakanda* section consists of those instructions on devotional service to God, which is found later in the *Vedanta-sutra*, the *Puranas* and other books.

The *Upanishads* are essentially presented for the continued spiritual progress of the individual. If the *Vedas* emphasize and primarily consist of worship to the demigods for material needs and only hint at the prospect of spiritual liberation, then the *Upanishads* start to explain how worldly attachments need to be renounced so we can surrender to God. The word *Upanishad* literally means to sit down (*shad*) near (*upa*) and below or at the feet with determination (*ni*). So it indicates that the student should sit near the feet of one's spiritual teacher and listen with determination to the teachings. Only through such absorption can one learn how to apply the teachings in practice. Sitting at the feet of the teacher is both a sign of respect and humility, but also exhibits a natural flow, like water, from something high to that which is lower. Thus the student becomes a natural receptacle for such knowledge. Another meaning of the word *shad* in *Upanishad* means to destroy. So the spiritual knowledge the student receives from the teacher destroys the ignorance of the true nature of the world and his own self. As one's ignorance is destroyed, enlightenment can follow. The *Upanishads* are a collection of 108 philosophical dissertations. The *Muktikopanishad* lists all 108. However, there are over one hundred additional compilations if you also count the lesser *Upanishads* that are not actually part of the primary group, making a total of well over two hundred. Out of all the *Upanishads*, the following eleven are considered to be the topmost: *Isa, Kena, Katha, Prasna, Mundaka, Mandukya, Taittiriya, Aitareya, Chandogya, Brihadaranyaka,* and *Svetasvatara*. The *Upanishads* were considered the secret and confidential knowledge of reality. They mainly focus on establishing the Absolute as nonmaterial and describe it as Brahman: the eternal, unmanifest reality, source, and ultimate shelter of everything. The Brahman is said to be incomprehensible because it is without material qualities or form. The secret to understanding Brahman according to the *Upanishads* is that they describe the Absolute as having no material qualities or material personality but consists of spiritual qualities. The comparisons used in the *Upanishads* can be somewhat confusing to the beginner of Vedic study, but they are easy to understand for one who has some understanding in this matter or who is self-realized. For example, when the *Upanishads* describe the Absolute as being unembodied, without veins, yet runs swifter than the mind, or as being able to walk yet does not walk, or as being within everything and yet outside of everything, how can we know what to think? Does the Absolute have any qualities that we can comprehend? These kinds of descriptions in the *Upanishads* are called indirect or contrary descriptions. These are used to indicate the spiritual nature of the Lord's qualities, meaning that he is not material nor confined to the rules of the material creation. An example of this is found in the *Svetashvatara Upanishad*, chapter 3, which explains,

The Supreme Lord does not have material hands and feet yet he is able to receive anything and go everywhere. He does not possess material eyes and yet he sees past, present, and future. He does not have material ears and yet he hears. He is the knower of everything, omniscient, but him no one can know. The self-realized and enlightened souls know him as the primeval Lord and Supreme Being.

The *Svetashvatara Upanishad* offers more of these kinds of descriptions, such as, *"He is having his faces, heads, and necks everywhere, yet he dwells in the cavity of the heart of all beings. He is omnipresent. Being the supreme Godhead, he is present everywhere encompassing all that exists and he is benevolent. With hands and feet everywhere, with eyes, heads and mouths everywhere, with ears everywhere, he stands encompassing all."* Another example is the *Isha Upanishad*: *"The Supreme Lord walks and does not walk. He is far away but he is very near as well. He is within everything, and yet he is outside of everything.* So the point is that the Absolute has spiritual legs to run or walk with and spiritual senses that are not limited like material senses.

One verse that clearly explains this is the following: *The Supreme Reality is far beyond this universe. He possesses no ephemeral form, but he is sat citananda, the embodiment of complete eternal and spiritual bliss. He is free from any ill. He is beyond the illusive world. He is full of all auspicious divine glories. Those who realize him as such and render unalloyed devotion to him become immortal, but others (who remain ignorant of him) have to undergo suffering through transmigration in the realm of maya, Sveta-shatara Upanishad.* Therefore, though the *Upanishads* generally refer to the Absolute in an impersonal way, they also begin to establish that the Supreme Reality has form, or, in other words, is a person, and that there is a divine abode, although the details of it are not always clearly provided therein. So as we go through the Vedic texts, we get clearer and clearer views of the nature of the Supreme Being. The *Isa Upanishad*, in particular, indicates that the supreme Absolute is both impersonal and personal. Other *Upanishads* describe the Absolute as, *"He who created the worlds,"* or, *"Who is luminous like the sun," "beyond darkness," "the eternal among eternals,"* etc. In fact, the basic method used in most *Upanishads*, as explained in the *Hayasirsa Pancharatra*, is to first present the Absolute Reality in an impersonal way and then present the personal aspects. Yet as we study the *Upanishads*, there are numerous references that go on to describe very clearly, in a direct manner, the spiritual nature and characteristics of the Supreme. The *Gopala Tapani Upanishad* has numerous verses which explain the nature of the Absolute Truth, such as the following verse, *"Sri Krishna is that Supreme Divinity, the Paramount Eternal Reality among all other sentient beings, and the fountain source of consciousness to all conscious beings. He is the only reality without a second, but as the supersoul, he dwells in the cave of the hearts of all beings and rewards them in accordance with their respective actions in life. Those men of intuitive wisdom who serve him with loving devotion surely attain the summum bonum, supreme goal of life. Whereas those who do not do so never gain this highest beatitude of their lives."*

Another verse from the *Gopala Tapani Upanishad* that further explains the nature of the Supreme is, *"Sri Krishna has got no birth and no old age, he is always in his adolescence without any change. He is ever most effulgently shining so gloriously more than the sun. He is fond of remaining with the divine cows of* Goloka *Vrindavana. He is eternally fond of being with the gopas, cowherd boys, as he feels pleasure tending the cows. He is the very object of the Vedas, he as the supersoul ever dwells in the heart of every living being, and he is the only sustainer of all. He is the beloved sweetheart of you all."*

Not only do the *Upanishads* provide explanations of the impersonal Brahman and personal Bhagavan realizations, but as we can see, they also speak of the Paramatma (Supersoul or Lord in the heart) realization. Especially in the *Katha, Mundaka,* and the *Svetasvatara Upanishads,* one can find statements explaining that within the heart of every individual in every species of life reside both the individual soul and the supersoul, the localized expansion of the Lord. It is described that they are like two birds sitting in the same tree of the body. The individual soul, which is called the *atma* or *jiva,* is engrossed in using the body to taste the fruits of various activities that result in pleasure and pain. The supersoul is simply witnessing the activities of the *jiva*. If, however, the *jiva* begins to tire of these constant ups and downs of material life and then looks toward his friend next to him, the supersoul, and seeks his help, the *jiva* soul can be relieved of all anxieties and regain his spiritual freedom. This freedom is the spiritual oneness shared by the *jiva* and Paramatma when the *jiva* enters into the spiritual atmosphere by submitting to the will of the Paramatma. This is achieved by the practice of yoga and by being guided by a proper spiritual master. It is not said that the individual soul loses his individuality, but both the jiva and Paramatma remain individuals. In any case, the *Upanishads* present a much clearer approach to understanding the ultimate reality than the four primary *Vedas*. We can provide a little more insight into the information found within the *Upanishads* by reviewing a few. The *Isha Upanishad* comes from the fortieth chapter of the *Shukla (white) Yajurveda*. It has only eighteen verses, but directly addresses the personality of God in the first verse. Through the eighteen verses, it gradually establishes that God has a personal form from which comes the great white Brahman effulgence. It explains that all opulence comes from God and that to try to enjoy such pleasures outside of the relationship with God is an illusion filled with suffering. Therefore, one should live life in such a way as to always remember God, and thus fulfill the real purpose of life so at the end one can constantly hold the vision of God within one's consciousness. When God removes his effulgence or spiritual rays, then the devotee can see the personal form of the Lord. The *Katha Upanishad* contains six chapters divided in two sections. Within it is the conversation between Nachiketa and Yamaraj, the lord of death. Within that conversation, Yamaraj establishes that due to ignorance and the desire to enjoy the material world, people continue to suffer in the cycle of birth and death, yet think they understand the real purpose of life. It is only in this human body that a person has the facility to realize God and escape the continued rounds of birth and death. Therefore, before the end of one's life, he or she should realize God in order to fully utilize this human birth. The *Mundaka Upanishad* contains six chapters in three sections. This gives the instruction from the *sage* Angira to Shaunaka about the nature of God and how to become realized. These instructions include how the early Brahmanas understood that the Vedic rituals only provided the means to acquire the luxuries of life, without being able to deliver one to God. Therefore, they gave them up for approaching a God realized saint, the only way one can learn how to surrender to the eternal Lord who is beyond all illusion of the universe. This is the God who cannot be understood by the Vedic impersonalistic philosophy, or intellectual meditation. The Lord is only realized when he reveals himself to one whose heart is full of devotion, after that person has been graced with such faithfulness by a saintly devotee. Then one can see the Lord as he is in full. The *Mandukya Upanishad* is another short *Upanishad* with only twelve verses. Herein it explains the impersonal aspect of God without going on to the personal traits. Here we find descriptions that can be confusing to those who are just beginning their investigation into Vedic philosophy, such as relating how the Absolute cannot be conceived by the mind, or contacted in any way. It has nothing that it can be compared to, and thus cannot be understood or spoken of, nor meditated upon because it is inconceivable. So from this *Upanishad,* based on the impersonal point of view, it would seem that there is little for us to understand about the Supreme. The *Svetasvatara Upanishad* is one of the most important. In its six chapters it elaborates on the more detailed characteristics of the soul, the Supreme Being, and the material nature, as well as the process for becoming spiritually realized. This is where we start to get deeper examples of the *paramatma*, the supersoul aspect of

God. It describes that God is the supreme pure consciousness from which all of creation manifests. And that God is realized when one becomes *lovingly absorbed in the Supreme*, which is the only way a person can cross the ocean of *maya*. It contains many relevant instructions and is one *Upanishad* that begins to take us much deeper into the understanding of the different aspects of the nature of God and the secrets of becoming God realized. The *Taittiriya Upanishad* goes into explaining more about the creative process of the material manifestation from the Brahman, and that the Brahman is from whom all souls emanate, and in Whom they enter at the time of the universal annihilation. That Brahman is eternally personified, by which he is knowable and reachable. Through that personified form, he expands bliss and divine love which we can experience through spiritual practice. This *Upanishad* is divided into three chapters called *Shiksha Valli*, *Brahmanand Valli*, and *Bhrigu Valli*. There are many other *Upanishads*, though they may be less prominent, that can be important to relating inner facts and secrets about the nature of God and how to realize him. So I'll mention a few. There is the *Krishna Upanishad* that directly reveals that the most divine form of bliss dwells in the supremacy of love of Lord Krishna. It elaborates that when Lord Krishna descended to earth in Braja Mandala, Vrindavana, the other eternal and divine personalities and powers also came with him in order to serve him and taste the sweetness of that *divine love*. The *Gopala Tapani Upanishad* goes much further in explaining things in this direction. It has only two chapters with a total of 172 verses. In the first chapter it explains that Lord Krishna is the absolute bliss. He is the supreme God and the embodiment of eternal life, knowledge and bliss. This is elaborated throughout the chapter. Chapter 2 explains how Lord Krishna is the supreme and most beautiful form of God. No other god or portion of this material creation can compare to his beauty. Therefore, it is recommended that we need to remember and adore him, by which we can experience his divine love, which is like an ocean of nectar. It is important to point out that the Sanskrit term for the experience of Krishna's divine love is *rasa*. It is the *Bhagavat Purana* that, in the Vedic literature, begins to explain the *rasalila* or bliss pastimes of Lord Krishna with his numerous associates. The word *rasa* is never used in connection with Lord Vishnu, Lord Shiva, Goddess Durga, or any of the other Vedic personalities in any of the *Upanishads*. That is because, though we may engage in respectful worship to these divinities, the pleasure pastimes wherein there is such a deep exchange of divine bliss and love is not to be found in anyone but Lord Krishna. Even the expansions of Lord Krishna, such as Lord Vishnu or Lord Rama, may be forms of unlimited bliss, but the deep exchanges of loving bliss with them do not have the potential that is found *within* Lord Krishna. Therefore, the conclusion is that Lord Krishna is the supreme personality in which is found all other forms of divinity and from whom comes the Absolute Truth and absolute loving bliss. The *Radhika Upanishad* explains this a little further. Therein it is described that only within Lord Krishna is there the *hladini* power, which is the pleasure or bliss potency. The other forms of the lord are but parts or expansions of the lord, and although they may be the same in power, they are lacking in the level of bliss potency that is found within Lord Krishna. This means that the supreme sweetness in loving exchanges is manifested from Lord Krishna. In this way, you have the sweet, sweeter, and sweetest levels of loving bliss established in the different levels of the spiritual reality, until it culminates from the Brahman and Vaikuntha on up to Goloka Vrindavana, the spiritual abode of Lord Krishna, or from the *brahmajyoti* to the Vishnu forms up to the supremacy of Sri Krishna. This is what is established by fully understanding the purport of the *Upanishads*. Another less prominent *Upanishad*, but one that is no less important, is the *Sri Chaitanya Upanishad* (*Chaitanyopanishad*), which comes from the ancient *Atharvaveda*. The *Chaitanyopanishad* is a short text with only nineteen verses. All of them are very significant. In this description there is not only the prediction of the appearance of Lord Chaitanya, but a description of his life and purpose, and the reasons why his process of spiritual enlightenment is so powerful and effective in this age of Kali Yuga. The *Chaitanyopanishad* explains how one day Pippalada, a son of Lord Brahma, approached his father and asked about how the sinful living entities in the age of Kali Yuga may be delivered. Lord Brahma told him to listen carefully, and he would give him a confidential description of what would happen in Kali Yuga. He explained that in Kali Yuga, the Supreme Being, whose form is completely transcendental and who is the all-pervading supersoul in the hearts of all living entities, will appear again in the Kali age. He will appear in the guise of the greatest devotee, with a golden complexion in his abode on the banks of the Ganges at Navadvipa. He will disseminate pure devotional service to the supreme. He will be known as Sri Chaitanya Mahaprabhu. Appearing in this golden form, the all-powerful Supreme Being—who is understood only by the most fortunate—who is the oldest, the original person, the original cause of the universe will spread spiritual bliss by the chanting of his own holy names. The Supreme Lord will chant a mantra consisting of the names of Hari, Krishna, and Rama (the

Hare Krishna *Mahamantra).* This mantra is the best of all mantras, and though difficult to understand, it can be understood by engaging in devotional service to the Supreme. This is the most confidential of secrets, and those who seriously desire to make progress in spiritual life and to cross the ocean of birth and death continually chant these names of the Supreme. Herein we find the assortment of information that can be found in the main *Upanishads*. For the most part, except for the more specialized and detailed *Upanishads* that were referred to at the end, they only briefly indicate the personal traits of the supreme personality and the divinity of Krishna and his abode. Mostly, they provide knowledge only up to the Brahman or Vaikuntha, not beyond. They express the nonmaterial, spiritual nature of God but do not know or present much information on the personality and pastimes of the Supreme Being. The end or conclusive result of knowledge in the *Upanishads* is to attain liberation from material existence. But what such liberation consists of is often left out. So information on the pastimes and nature of the abode of God and the spiritual domain is generally absent. This is the case with most all of the s*hruti* texts, which consist of the four divisions of the *Vedas*: Samhita *Brahmana, Aranyakas,* and *Upanishads.* Once you get beyond the rituals and methods for acquiring material needs by worship of the Vedic demigods, the s*hruti* texts primarily contain knowledge of the futility of material existence, the temporary nature of the material creation, the bondage of the *jiva* souls in this existence of birth and death, and the spiritual nature of the individual and the Supreme Being. In parts, they may also describe that the goal of life is liberation from this material manifestation and the need to return to spiritual existence through the understanding of *karma*, spiritual knowledge, renunciation and devotion to God (*bhakti*). However, they are unaware of much beyond this, or at least the finer details. They do not deliver information about the bliss of spiritual activities and the pastimes of Goloka Vrindavana, the most intimate and confidential abode of the Lord who is a spiritual being, a personality. Because of this basic deficiency, additional information is supplied elsewhere, which must be sought and understood. As we can see, this is a progressive ladder of education, in which case one should not stop with the *Upanishads*. Aside from the *Upanishads*, there are also the *Upavedas*. These are the *Artha Veda* (science of economics and sociology), the *Dhanur Veda* (the science of defense, war, and politics), the *Gandharva Veda* (art of music, dancing, and singing), and *Ayurveda* (the holistic medical science). These are smaller compositions, each are attached to one of the four main *samhitas* (namely the *Rig, Yajur, Sama,* and *Atharva* respectively). Unfortunately, most of these compositions are difficult to find, except for the *Ayurveda*, the majority of which is still available but not all of its original text. These are a part of the eighteen principal branches of Vedic knowledge, which, according to the *Vishnu Purana*, are listed with their sources as the six *Ve-dangas*: the four *Vedas*, the six *Angas* (or subsidiary portions of the *Vedas*), viz., *Siksha*, rules of reciting the prayers, the accents, and tones to be observed; *Kalpa*, ritual; *Vyakarana*, grammar; *Nirukta*, glossarial comment; *Chandas*, metre; and *Jyotish*, astronomy; with *Mimamsa*, theology; *Nyaya*, logic; *Dharma*, the institutes of law; and the *Puranas*, constitute the fourteen principal branches of knowledge. Or they are considered as eighteen with the addition of these four: the *Ayurveda*, medical science as taught by Lord Dhanvantari; *Dhanur-Veda*, the science of archery or military arms taught by

Bhrigu; *Gandharva Veda*, or drama and the arts of music, dancing, etc., of which the Muni Bharata was the author; and the *Artha Shastram*, or science of government, as laid down first by Brihaspati. (*Vishnu Purana*, book 3, chapter 6)

To briefly explain some of the branches mentioned above: *Vyakarana* is the science of Sanskrit grammar. This is presently based on the Panini grammar, since the other ancient forms or books are extinct. The Panini system, which has some four thousand *sutras*, is said to have been inspired by Lord Shiva when he once played on his small *damru* drum from which came fourteen separate sounds. Those vibrations inspired Panini, who then explained the science of Sanskrit grammar. These vibrations were said to be originally in the mysterious formula of the *Maheshvara Sutra*. This *Sutra* is said to contain all sounds arranged in an order that holds the key to all structure of language. Panini also provided the *Dhatu Path*, which is a dictionary of the root Sanskrit words. Then he gave the *Unadi Sutras* to describe how the words in the original Vedic *samhitas* (the four *Vedas*) were formed, which can provide the means of understanding the real definition of the words in the *samhita* mantras. Without this, it is easy for a person to mistranslate the real meaning or purpose of the Vedic mantras. *Nirukta* provides the explanations of the Vedic words. It is used along with the *Nighantu*, which is a collection of Vedic words with their basic explanations. These are used with the *Vyakarana* to understand the exact meaning of Sanskrit words to make sure the Vedic *samhita* mantras are not misunderstood. *Siksha* is the science of correct pronunciation of Vedic mantras, such as intonation, duration, and the accent on a word or syllable. This will determine how one "sings" each mantra. Differences in the pronunciation of a mantra can also change its meaning, and the outcome of the ritual. That is one of the reasons why the old Vedic rituals are no longer recommended for this day and age. The problem is that this is difficult to learn and almost all books on the topic have become lost.

Chandas is the science of correctly emphasizing the meter of the Vedic verses according to the division or parts and letters, and the correct pronunciation of the words. The Vedic mantras are also named according to its parts. For example, the *Anushtup Chand* is a mantra of four parts in one stanza, and with thirty-two letters. Yet if it has thirty-one letters in four parts, it is called *Brihati Chand*, and so on. *Jyotish* is the science of Vedic astrology. This was used for a couple of reasons. Primarily it was for establishing the correct position of the stars and planets at certain times, such as one's birth, and their effects for predicting one's future life. It was also for calculating the best times to begin special activities, such as Vedic rituals. There were many books on *Jyotish*, but most have now become lost, leaving but several left to study.

The *Artha Sastram* is said to have been established first by Brihaspati, but was written most recently by Kautilya in the fourth century BC for the king, Chandragupta Maurya. It is the science of government and economics that takes credit for some of the principles of corporate management that have gained popularity today, such as using *Prabhu Shakti* (vision), *Mantra Shakti* (mission), and *Utsah Shakti* (motivation). The *Mimamsa*, *Dharma*, and *Nyaya* are parts of the Vedic Sutras, which is explained next. When it comes to the Mimamsa, there is the *Purva Mimamsa* and the *Uttar Mimamsa*. First there is the *Purva Mimamsa* that was written by the sage Jaimini who was a student of *Vyasadeva* about five thousand years ago.

The *Uttara Mimamsa* is the *Brahma* or *Vedanta* sutras, which is discussed soon. *Mimamsa* means solutions through critical examination, and was originally expounded by Jaimini in the twelve chapters of his *Mimamsa sutra*. It clarifies the Vedic principles so a person can focus on the ways for attaining a good life now and in the next. This system was traditionally called *Purva Mimamsa*, representing the early revered thought. This is in relation to the study of Vedanta since *Mimamsa* was considered the preliminary understanding of Vedanta philosophy. On the other hand, Vedanta is also called *Uttara Mimamsa*, meaning the conclusion and higher teachings of the Mimamsa philosophy, because the Vedas are regarded as self evident scriptures that reveal divine knowledge. The Mimamsa system emphasizes the importance of action in terms of ritual, worship, and duty or *Dharma* as the means of reaching liberation from *karma* and the cycle of repeated birth and death. It explains the essential Vedic issues and describes the eternal nature of the Vedic texts as part of the same spiritual energy as God, which are manifested on earth through the minds of the great sages. It then continues to clarify the accurate use of the Vedic mantras for the attainment of happiness and material facility.

Mimamsa is basically a systematized code of rules for the Vedic rituals and worship used along with the *Vedas* and explains the purpose and meaning of the rituals. It is especially meant to help householders regulate and spiritualize their daily lives, while Vedanta is meant more for those who had grown tired of materialistic existence and are ready to retire and seriously engage in spiritual pursuits.

Dharma is considered to be those moral activities that harmonize individual life with cosmic life. The *Nyaya Sutra* presents the Vedic system of logic as established by the *sage Gautama*. This was written in a question and answer format, like many of the Vedic *Sutras*.

Nyaya is a school of logic which regards doubt as a prerequisite for philosophical inquiry. All other Indian systems of philosophy use the Nyaya system of logic as a foundation for reasoning and debate. The five principles of the Nyaya system are: (1) to present the proposition, (2) the reason for presenting the proposition, (3) an example of it, showing that it is realistic or unrealistic, depending on the instance, (4) apply the example of the proposition presented, and (5) establish the conclusion of the proposition. The ultimate purpose of the Nyaya system, which is closely linked to the Vaisheshika system, is to use this process of logic to establish the ultimate truth, or God, the Supreme Reality, and to show the spiritual platform is all that is truly desirable and not the temporary material creation. It is meant to help one achieve liberation from karma and material existence by properly understanding reality, or the difference between matter and spirit. Nyaya accepts that the only way to liberation is to obtain knowledge of the external world and understand its relationship with the mind and self. Through logical criticism, one can discriminate between truth and illusion and, applying such understanding in daily life, rid oneself of suffering and attain liberation. Additionally, this system of logic was developed to prove the validity of its principles by analysis and argument to counter the criticism of the Buddhists, Jains, and Charvakas. However, the Nyaya system was empirical and mostly relied on perception, inference, comparison, and testimony as its means of acquiring knowledge. The *Vaisheshika Sutra*, written in a question and answer format, was the first work written on this philosophy by Kanada. Prasastapada later wrote a definitive commentary on this *sutra* entitled *Svartha Dharma Samgraha*. The name Vaisheshika comes from *vishesha*, which means uniqueness or particularity. Therefore, the Vaisheshika system is a study of the uniqueness and qualities of existence, such as the elements, atoms, their interactions, as well as the soul. But it accepts only two independent sources of knowledge, which are perception and inference. It is a *sutra* that helps show the futility of life in the temporary worlds of *maya*, and the need for understanding God and to become free from all *karma* so that liberation can follow. However, the knowledge within this sutra is unnecessary if one already knows that understanding God and regaining one's devotional love is the real goal of life. *The Vaisheshka Sutra* contained several ideas: (1) that everything is composed of atoms bearing the qualities of either earth, water, light, or air; (2) that the individual souls are eternal and pervade a material body for a time; (3) there are nine basic elements, consisting of earth, water, light, air, ether, time, space, soul, and mind, which are all eternal in the form of energy; and (4) there are seven categories of experience, which are substance, quality, activity, generality, particularity, inherence, and nonexistence.

However, God is not mentioned in the *sutra*, but later commentators included knowledge of God to complete the system. Vaisheshika attempted to integrate philosophical theories with moral and spiritual attitudes or *dharma* which would lead people to good in this life and the next. However, it did not bring the Supreme Being to the point of ultimate reality, but as merely an agent of release from *karma* and repeated birth and death. Therefore, the *Vaisheshika* philosophy is not complete in its understanding of the Absolute Truth or of material nature. The Vaisheshika theory is that merely by interactions between atoms, the elements are formed, and thus, the world and all objects within appear. However, this is refuted by the *Vedanta sutras*. For example, if atoms are simply inert matter, then atomic combinations could not properly take place without some higher directional force. The Vaisheshikas say this force is the unseen principle but fail to explain fully what it is, where it resides, or how it works. They also say that atoms and relationships between the atoms of the elements as earth, water, air, etc, are eternal, but this would mean that any form composed of atoms would also be eternal, such as the material world and all that is in it. However, anyone can see that this is not the case since everything is always changing and breaking apart. Even the Vaisheshikas accept the fact that all bodies and forms composed of atoms are temporary. In this way, we can recognize the contradictions in the atomic theory of the Vaisheshikas, which is therefore unacceptable.

The *Sankhya* philosophy is another system. The principal aim is to analyze the distinctions between matter and spirit. The study of the twenty-four material elements was originally developed as a complex science by Lord Kapila, as elaborated in *Srimad-Bhagava-tam*. But later, there was another Kapila who presented an atheistic Sankhya system. Therefore, in other schools of this system, the existence of God is considered irrelevant. This is because the universe is regarded as a system of cause and effect. In other words, the cause of the universe is that which is eternal but ever changing, or *prakriti*, the ever changing material energy. God is eternal and nonchanging, so within this atheistic view of Sankhya, it is considered that God cannot be the cause of the universe. Obviously, there are limitations in this analysis, such as not defining where *prakriti* came from and how could *prakriti*, which is inert form the material universe without any guidance, and so on. So gradually, there were additional arguments that again led to an acceptance of God in the philosophy of Sankhya.

The original Sankhya system, as explained in *Srimad-Bhagavatam* by Lord Kapila, acknowledges matter and spirit as two separate principles of reality. Thus, genuine Sankhya introduces a dualistic philosophy more developed than the previous three systems discussed so far. Sankhya analyzed such factors as *purusha* and *prakriti* (spirit and matter), the creation and development of matter through excitation of the *purusha*, how the world evolved, how the modes of nature operate and affect us, *how ahankara (false ego) causes our identification with matter* and bondage to the material world, the five organs of action and five senses of perception, the subtle elements, the gross elements, etc. The goal of this system is to understand that the real self is eternal and free, but because of ignorance the soul identifies with what is temporary and therefore suffers. Through this kind of analysis of the material world it is expected that one will realize the difference between matter and spirit and attain freedom from false identification. After this stage is attained, release from existence in the material world is reached through spiritual training, *meditation* on the real self and superself, and the practice of yoga. Yoga is the next system, which is the application of the Sankhya system. Sankhya is the theory, and yoga is the practice. Yoga, which is essentially theistic, *was* known many years before Patanjali. Although he is often given the credit for it, he merely codified it in his Yoga Sutras. The complete system of yoga is very complex and has many steps to it, each of which must be perfected before one can go on to the next step. The purpose of yoga is to suspend the flickering nature and internal dictations of the mind. Yoga is also to attain relief from the pain that exists from such things as ignorance, which brings attachment, which then leads the way to fear and hatred, as well as the fear of death. The practice of yoga and renunciation is for bringing freedom from such pains and suffering. Although the basis of this system may be quite popular, few people can actually reach the higher levels of self realization through this process in this day and age. The different levels of this process and yoga systems are briefly explained further. The other subsidiary portions of the *Vedas* previously mentioned in the *Vedangas* have additional texts that further explain that section of Vedic knowledge. For example, the *Kalpa-sutras,* which elaborate on the many kinds of rituals, are divided into four kinds, namely the *Shrauta sutras*, *Grihya sutras*, *Dharma sutras*, and the *Shulba sutras*. The *Shrauta sutras* explain the rituals the priests engage in, and the details of performing a Vedic *yajna*, or ceremony, according to the particular branch of the *Veda* with which it is connected. It covers the large and royal rituals performed by kings, such as the *ashvamedha* or *rajasuya*, to the ordinary ones performed by a family, such as the *agnishtoma*, *agnihotra*, or the *pitri yajna* for the dead relatives. The *Grihya sutras* describes the general and ritualistic social traditions that are usually observed by house holders for their upliftment. These include such things as the performance of daily worship, study of scripture, or installing a deity in a temple. Also, how to greet a guest, do rituals for moving into a new house, or timely *samskaras* for giving a name to a child, or the ritual for a child's first hair cutting, a youth's acceptance of a Vedic order, or the marriage ceremony. The *Dharma sutras* deal with the different disciplines or duties of a person, from common individuals up to the king. This includes duties of people in the four orders of life (from birth up to renunciation, or *brahmacari* student to *sannyasa*), along with duties of a man to his family and society, or duties of a married couple to each other and their children, or duties of a king to his subordinates.

Vedic mathematics is found in the *Shulba Sutras*, which means "codes of the rope" since particular lengths of rope were used to make exact measurements.

The *Shulba sutras* had 1180 branches and give mathematical details on size and shape of altars for the fire rituals and the place where such ceremonies would take place. The mathematical codes are said to have been compiled from the eighth to the fifth century BC, however such codes probably existed far earlier than this. It is figured that the original Indian mathematical developments arose from the needs of their religious ceremonies that required altars of precise measurement. This started to gain significance when the sages began to emphasize the use of external processes of worship and ritual as an additional means to attain internal awareness and spiritual progress. In other words, they were not interested in math outside of what it could do for them spiritually. The *Shulba Sutras* show the earliest forms of algebra as used by the Vedic priests. The *Shulba Sutras* were only a portion of the broader system of mathematics found in the *Kalpa Sutras*. These consisted of arithmetic and algebra as well as geometry. In fact, geometrical instruments dating back to 2500 BC have been found in the Indus Valley, which was also a part of Vedic society. The Pythogorean Theorem was already existing in the Shulba Sutras before Pythagoras presented it. This means he may have only learned of it through his travels in India rather than inventing it himself. It was the Vedic system that developed the decimal system of tens, hundreds, thousands, etc., and how to take the remainder of one column of numbers over to the next.

When I say the Vedas are more science than religion, I am not exaggerating; in India they did turn Vedas into Hinduism. Hinduism is the predominant and indigenous religions of India. They did try to turn Vedas into only religion, but in reality, Vedas are basically the science of the soul (during many centuries, Vimanas were pretty much hidden from main streams only few handle such knowledge) mankind has been doing this for thousands of years. We also can mention the historical book, the Bible, which is not scientific but, otherwise, historical. (*Science* from Latin *scientia*, meaning "knowledge" is a systematic enterprise that builds and organizes knowledge.)

The numeral system of nine numbers and a zero (0) made calculations very easy. Without the invention and use of zero (0), many of the mathematical advancements that have been made in the West would not have been possible. These numbers were developed from the Brahmi script and became popular after AD 700, spreading into Arabia. They became known as the Arabic numerals because the Europeans, who had adopted them, got them from the traveling Arabians. Yet the Arabians called them "Indian figures" (*AlArqan AlHindu*) because they had received them from India. Because of this, it was called the India art (*hindisat*). Thus, *the system of math that we all use today had its start in Vedic India.* Further developments in mathematics in India by its mathematicians, such as Brahmagupta (seventh century), Mahavira (ninth century), and Bhaskara (twelfth century) in such areas as algebra and trigonometry were not known in Europe until the seventeenth and eighteenth centuries. In fact, many of the great inventions made in Europe that we take for granted today, would have been impossible if they had been stuck with their cumbersome Roman numerals, and without the advanced system of mathematics that came from India. The *Anukramanika* is another book in the same category as these *sutras* and relates the contents of the *Vedas*. It consists of 1180 books for the 1180 Vedic branches. It lists all of the Vedic gods and their associated mantras, and all the sages who composed them. So this works like a summary of the Vedic books. Beyond these are many other texts that include the *Sraddhakalpa, Pitrimedhasutras, Parisistas, Prayogas, Karikas,* etc., all of which deal only with Vedic rituals. A later text that also deals with the Vedic rituals is the *Rig vidhana* by the sage Shaunaka. This book gives explanations on the usage of many of the verses or hymns in the *Rig-Veda*. The precise chanting of particular verses produces specific magical or quick results, such as overcoming one's enemies, getting rid of disease, protecting oneself from ghosts, and many other things. The *Rigvidhana* indicates which verses, and the procedure if necessary, to be used to accomplish their various effects.

Additional topics, such as alchemy, are also dealt with, or architecture as found in the Sthapatya veda, or erotics as found in the Kama Sutra. India also had a long agricultural heritage that went back to before 3700 BC, and had the first written texts on the topic. One of the oldest books is the *Krishi Parashara* (c. 400 BC), which means Agriculture by Parashara. This has been translated by the Asian Agri History Foundation in Secunderabad, India. This book gives lists of tools to be used, ways of predicting rain by using basic astrology with climate conditions, methods of good farming management for the high yield of crops, management of cattle, along with advice on seed collection and storage, etc. Another text on agriculture was the *Kashyapiyakrishisukti* by Kashyapa (c. AD 700-800). This describes the means of producing certain crops, cattle management, soil properties, laying out gardens, means of irrigation, marketing, ways of support from the government, as well as mining, and even a personal code of conduct for farmers. The Vrikshayurveda (The Science of Plant Life) by Surapala was another book that appeared later (c. AD 1000).

This dealt with the application of Ayurveda to various kinds of trees. However, it also contained knowledge of raising orchards, seed management, selection of soil, ways of irrigation, finding groundwater, using fertilizers, dealing with plant diseases, and so on. These books recommend practical ways of efficient farming while preserving the world's resources and environment, along with the means by which humanity can achieve the essential aims of life, such as *dharma*, *artha*, *kama*, and *moksha* (religion, economic development, sensual fulfillment, and liberation through spiritual advancement) which are all things that we should still consider today. The *Smritis* were additional books that included those of many ancient authors, such as the *Manusamhita*, the famous Vedic law book, and *Yagyavalkya Smriti*, *Parashar Smriti*, and those of Brihaspati, Daksha, Gautama, Yama, Angira, Pracheta, Yogeshwa-ra, Atri, Vishnu, and several others. There were also the *UpaSmritis* (smaller books) of Na-rada, Pulaha, Garga, Pulastya, Shaunaka, Kratu, Baudhayana, Jatukarna, Vishvamitra, Pi-tamaha, Jabali, Skanda, Kashyapa, Vyasa, Sanatkumara, Janaka, Vashishta, Bharadwaj and others. Most anyone who has done a fair amount of Vedic study will recognize these names, *but most of these books are now unavailable.* These *Smritis*, especially like the *Ma-nusamhita*, explained the codes and laws or disciplines of proper conduct, and the consequences or recommended penances for bad or evil behavior. They prescribe the kind of fasting or charity or austerity one should perform for curing oneself of various sins, and what a person could expect if he was not relieved of such karmic reactions. However, some of the rules and laws it presents were meant for a much more conservative and stricter day and age. Thus, they are not as applicable in these modern times. The first three *Smritis* mentioned above are the most important. However, their content is mostly for attaining good results in the next life or for attaining heaven or celestial opulence and avoiding "hell (not a pleasurable life)." These generally do not provide the means for attaining complete liberation or God realization, although the *Manusamhita* does include such things as a description of proper behavior between guru and disciple. Nonetheless, just as with the *Upanishads*, there are some *Smritis* that do relate the more confidential aspects of how to reach the perfection of life and attain liberation and God realization. For example, the *Smriti* of Sanatkumara,

The *Sri Sanat kumara Samhita*, is still available today and has over 321 verses. It is said to be connected with the *Skanda Purana*. It starts by describing the unfortunate characteristics of the people in this age of Kali Yuga, and then goes on to explain the need for all people, from the lowest to the highest, to take shelter of the holy names of Hari, Krishna, as the only way to attain the Lord. (By means of love and meditation, it is considered to be the most noble way to attain God). It then prescribes two mantras that are most effective for this purpose, and explains how to chant them. It later goes into some detail in describing the sweet pastimes of Lord Krishna and his associates in the spiritual world. In this way, this specialized and rare *Smriti* describes the way for God realization and the most secret of secrets for complete liberation from material existence. After the above-mentioned *sutras*, we now come to the *Vedanta sutras*. When it comes to Vedanta, many commentaries on it revolve around the Brahman. The Brahman generally means the all-pervading self-existent power. The word "*Brahman*" is based on the root word "*brah*," which means vastness, power, or expansion. It also denotes the Supreme Being, as well as the *atman*, the living being, who, when freed from the body, becomes situated on the level of Brahman, or the spiritual nature. The concept of the Brahman was, for the most part, first elaborated in the *Upanishads*. Therein we begin to find descriptions from which our understanding of it grows. It is described as invisible, ungraspable, eternal, without qualities, and the imperishable source of all things. (*Mundaka Upanishad* 1.1.67) It is explained that Shankara's *advaita* doctrine was based on the famous passage in the *Chandogya Upanishad* (6.10.3), *tat tvam asi*, meaning "That thou art." He taught that "thou and that" were not to be regarded as object and subject, but as identical, without difference (*abheda*), like the real self (*atman*). Thus, anything that was variable, like the body, mind, intellect, and ego are objects of knowledge and not the *atman*. These concepts were more fully explained on the basis of the *Vedanta sutras*. The *Vedanta sutras* are a systematization of *sutras* or codes for understanding Vedic knowledge. As you know, they are short codes that are later to be explained by the spiritual master, guru or spiritual authority. By themselves, without further explanations, it is not easy to fathom their depths. So it is these commentaries that contain the additional information about such things as the Brahman. Vedanta means the conclusion of the *Veda* or end of all knowledge. Vedanta is also known as *Uttara Mimamsa*, or later examination, and is a companion to the *Purva Mima-msa*, or preliminary examination. The *Purva Mimamsa* deals with the early portions of the *Vedas* and the *Uttara Mimamsa* deals with the latter portions. The Vedic tradition, unlike other religions and philosophies, is rooted in such remote antiquity that its origin cannot be fully traced. The Vedic literature explains that it exists in the form of eternal spiritual vibrations and is present both within and outside the universal creation. Vedanta has been the most influential of the seven main systems of Eastern philosophy. Though the name Vedanta is often taken to indicate the impersonal, nondual, or Mayavada school of thought, it is essentially dualistic theism; but various commentaries have interpreted it to mean different things. It was the *SarirakaBhasya* commentary by Shankara that established the Vedanta as a nondualistic philosophy, meaning that the ultimate reality is but one. In this regard, the Brahman and the Atman (individual souls) are identical, and the Brahman is the Absolute Reality from which everything manifests and back into which everything merges. This interpretation has gained much respect and influence, but is not the only or ultimate viewpoint of Vedic literature, as will be explained.

The *Vedanta sutras* are like short, condensed bits of information used as reminders for the spiritual master in his discussions on Vedic philosophy with a student or disciple. Each line, therefore, is meant to be elaborated upon by the spiritual master for the understanding of the student. Vedanta means "the end of knowledge," or the final conclusion of the Vedic philosophy. The *Vedanta sutras* are also called the *Brahma sutra, Sariraka, Vyasa sutra, Vedanta darshana, Uttaramimamsa,* as well as *Badarayana sutra.* Vyasa and Badarayana are two names for the same person who is considered to be the author and compiler of the major portions of Vedic literature. The *Vedanta sutras* are divided into four chapters with four divisions each. In each division the theme within is stated, reasons for it are given, examples are supplied to uphold the presented facts, the theme is then explained further for clearer understanding, and finally authorized quotations from the *Vedas* are supplied to support it. In this way, the information is given in a format meant to show the authenticity and reliability of the Vedic viewpoint. The first two chapters discuss how the material world manifested from the Supreme and the relationship between the living entity and the Supreme. The third chapter explains how one engages in the prescribed duties to perform and how to act according to the loving relationship we have with the Lord. The fourth chapter describes the result of such devotional service (or *bhakti*), which is ultimately to attain liberation or return to the spiritual world. The first verse of the *Vedanta sutras* states, "athato brahma jijnasa," which means, "Now is the time to inquire about the Absolute Truth." Why is it time? Because we are presently in the human form of life and should utilize it properly since only in the human form do we have the intelligence and facility to be able to understand spiritual reality. In animal forms, the living entities cannot understand such things because they do not have the brainpower. So we should not waste this human form of life by pursuing only the animalistic propensities, such as eating, sleeping, mating and defending. Therefore, the *Vedanta sutras* begin by stating that now is the time for us to understand the Absolute Truth. The *Vedanta sutras*, however, being written only in codes, can be somewhat vague and requires a commentary to elaborate and explain the aphorisms. Practically speaking, some of the codes are fairly unclear for anyone who is not experienced in Vedic philosophy. And since Vedanta comprises the purport of the *Upanishads,* which contain knowledge of both the personal and impersonal aspects of the Absolute, which commentary on the *Vedanta sutras* you read can make a big difference. Some commentaries way toward the impersonal understanding of the Absolute, while other commentaries sway toward the personal realizations. Obviously, to reach a mature understanding in this regard, we need to comprehend both of these viewpoints. In fact, it is stated that unless one understands all the features of the Absolute Truth, namely, the impersonal Brahman, the localized Paramatma, or supersoul, and ultimately the supreme personality of God, Bhagavan, or Krishna, one's knowledge is imperfect. After studying the previous portions of the Vedic literature, only when we arrive at this *Brahma sutras* or *Vedanta sutras* of Srila Vyasadeva do we find an emphasis on doing *bhakti yoga*, or devotional activities, for realizing God. This means that God is ultimately the supreme person from whom there is the imminent loving exchange that can be attained by lovingly surrendering to him. That devotion and emotional absorption in God is the process for becoming free from the illusory attraction and attachments to the material world. This paves the way for genuine liberation from worldly existence. There have been many commentaries written on the *Vedanta sutras*. The most influential were by such famous *acharyas* as Shankara, Bhaskara, Ramanuja, Nimbarka, Vallabha, Madhva, and Baladeva. So let us review a few of these to get a better view of the development of the *advaita* and *dvaita* philosophies. Let me point out here that the Vedic process has a unique system of checks and balances found nowhere else. This involves what you could call the three S system, namely *sadhu* (saintly devotees), *shastra* (Vedic texts) and spiritual master or *acharya*. If you ever want to know if you are taking the right path and are not being misled, you use this system. This means that any truth that you are given must be verified by these three sources of guru, *shastra* and *sadhus*. Even if a guru tells you something that cannot be verified in the *shastra* or by other *sadhus*, then it should be questioned or taken with caution. *Sadhu, shastra,* and spiritual master must all verify the points in order to be considered authentic and truth. So now we are going to read about what some of the most prominent *acharyas* or spiritual authorities have said about what the ultimate reality is and how to understand it. One of the most influential was Shankara (509-477 BC, though others have said AD 788-820). He was a follower of Shiva, born of a South Indian *brahmana* family in the town of Kaladi, on the banks of the Periyar River. His father's name was Shivaguru, and he lost his father at a young age. When he was only eight years old he finished his studies of all the scriptures and took sannyasa from Govinda who stayed on the banks of the Narmada and was a disciple of Gaudapada, the author of *Mandukyakarika*, a commentary on the *Mandukya Upanishad*. Not long after that he left for Varanasi, and then for Badarikashrama in the Himalayas. There he stayed until his twelfth year. While there he wrote his commentary on the *Brahma sutra*, as well as on ten *Upanishads* and *Bhagavad Gita*. He continued to travel and preach and made many disciples. He left this world at the early age of thirty-three. He established four main *maths*, or schools of study. These were at Dwaraka in the west, Jagannatha Puri in the east, Badrinatha in the north, and Shringeri in the south. These have records of their original establishment and list all of the successive *acharyas* who followed from the time of Shankaracharya. One of these lists, such as the one displayed at the Kamakoti Shankara Math in Kanchipuram, date back to 477 BC, thus dating earlier than the time of Christ. Shankaracharya's two major works are the *Vividacudamani* and *Sarirakabhasya*. When Shankara appeared, Buddhism and anti-Vedic thought had spread throughout India because it had been patronized by Emperor Asoka in the third century BC, and the followers of Buddhism had given up the *Vedas*. The Buddhist philosophy establishes that the material creation is the only manifestation of the Absolute Truth, which itself is temporary and brought on by egoistic desires. It is asserted that these desires must be eliminated for one to enter back into the void. The void itself is said to be all that is real and eternal, and the source from which everything manifests.

Shankara's purpose, therefore, was to reform and purify religious life by reestablishing the authority of the Vedic scriptures. His interpretation of the *Vedas* are known as *advaita* or nondualistic because he taught that the individual *jiva* or soul is identical with God, and that there is ultimately no variety, no individuality or personality in spiritual existence. The individuality of both the Supreme Being and the *jiva*, according to him, is false. In order for Shankara to teach like this, he had to ignore the many statements in the Vedic literature which assert that the Absolute Truth is the Supreme Person and the *jivas* are his subordinate parts. Therefore, by word jugglery, he developed a twofold theory that Brahman consists of the pure impersonal Brahman, and that any incarnation of God within this universe is simply a manifestation of that Brahman. This was a complete rejection of the personalistic teachings found in some of the Vedic literature, such as *Bhagavad Gita*, and in this way he differed with all orthodox Vedic schools at the time. Like Buddha, he also refused to answer questions about the origin of the cosmos and said that *maya*, the illusory energy, was inexplicable.

This Mayavada philosophy teaches that the material world is false and the impersonal. Brahman, or great white light or spiritual force, is the ultimate truth. One merges back into the Brahman, where there exist no activities or spiritual characteristics, after giving up the ego or bodily consciousness. Therefore, we find that impersonalists generally do not study the *Vedas* beyond the *Vedanta sutras* because as we progress through the Vedic literature up to the *Puranas*, it becomes more specific about the personal characteristics of the

Absolute Truth and the individual nature of the *jiva* souls, which contradicts the impersonal view point. We must point out that some spiritual authorities say that Shankaracharya was an incarnation of Lord Shiva.

Who had been ordered by the Supreme Lord to cheat the atheists. The *Shiva Purana* quotes the Supreme Lord as ordering Shiva: "In Kali Yuga mislead the people in general by propounding imaginary meanings from the *Vedas* [Vedic literature] to bewilder them," or *dvaparadau yuge bhutva, kalaya manushadishu svagamaih kalpitais tvam ca, janan madvimukhan kuru.*

The *Padma Purana* also says that Lord Shiva would descend as a brahmana sannyasi and teach Mayavada philosophy in the verse, *mayavada ashat shastram prachchanna boudhyam uchyate moya ebe godidam devi kalou brahmana murtina.*

To do this, Shankara gave up the direct method of Vedic knowledge and presented an indirect meaning which actually covered the real goal of Vedanta. This is confirmed in the *Padma Purana* where Lord Shiva addresses his wife, Parvati: *shrinu devi pravaksyami, tamasani yathakramam yesham shravanamatrena, patityam jnaninam api apartham shrutivakyanam, darshayal lokagarhitam karmasvarupatyajyatvam, atraca pratipadyate sarvakarmaparibhramsan, naiskarmyam tatra cocyate paratmajivayor aikyam, mayatra pratipadyate.*

> My dear wife, hear my explanations of how I have spread ignorance through Mayavada philosophy. Simply by hearing it even an advanced scholar will fall down. In this philosophy which is certainly very inauspicious for people in general, I have misrepresented the real meaning of the

Vedas and recommended that one give up all activities in order to achieve freedom from karma. In this Mayavada philosophy I have described the jivatma and Paramatma to be one and the same.

The *Padma Purana*, in the quote that follows, describes how Lord Shiva tells his wife, Parvati, that he would appear in Kali Yuga to teach the impersonalistic philosophy, which is impious and merely a covered form of Buddhism. Yet as explained next, there was a purpose for it. *Mayavadam asacchastram, pracchannam bauddham ucyate mayaiva kalpitam devi, kalau brahmana rupini brahmanas caparam rupam, nirgunam vaksyate maya sarvasv-am jagato'py asya, mohanartham kalau yug vedante tu mahashastre, mayavadam avaidikam mayaiva vaksyate devi, jagatam nashakaranat.*

> The mayavada philosophy is impious. It is covered buddhism. my dear Parvati, in the form of a brahmana in kali yuga I teach this imagined mayavada philosophy. In order to cheat the atheists I mislead them by describing the supreme Lord to be without any personal form or qualities.

Herein, Lord Shiva himself points out that to believe God has no form is not accurate and is equal to atheism. Even though this Mayavada philosophy was not good for pious people to hear because it would sway them toward an impersonalistic viewpoint, we should note that Shankara's philosophy was just right for the time and circumstance. The Buddhists, who had spread throughout India and neglected the *Vedas*, believed in neither a soul nor a God and that, ultimately, the essence of everything is the nothingness or void wherein lies *nirvana*, or freedom from all suffering. So considering how the Buddhists had followed a philosophy of what would generally be considered atheism for hundreds of years and would never have accepted a viewpoint which advocated a supreme personal God, Shankara's was the only philosophy they would have considered. It was like a compromise between atheism and theism, but Shankara used portions of Vedic knowledge as the basis of his arguments. In this way, as Shankara traveled throughout India his arguments prevailed. Thus, Buddhism bowed and Vedic culture was brought back to prominence. Therefore, his purpose was accomplished, so much so that his *Sarirakabhasya* is considered the definitive rendition of Vedanta even to the present day. Several times, however, Shankara revealed his true beliefs, that he was actually a devotee of Lord Krishna. For example, in the first verse of his *Vividacudamani*, he explains that it is Krishna himself who is the source of the supreme bliss and the divine master to whom he offers obeisance. Furthermore, in his birthplace of Kaladi, there is a temple near the *samadhi* tomb of his mother that has a deity of Lord Krishna that was installed by Shankara himself. So why would he give his mother the facility to worship Krishna if he was also not in favor of such a view?

Also, in his *Gitabhasya*, the first verse explains that Narayana (another incarnation of Lord Krishna), or Bhagavan, is transcendental to the material creation. In *Bhagavad Gita with the Commentary of Sri Sankaracarya*, Dinkar Vishnu Gokhale establishes that Shankara writes in his *Meditations on the Bhagavad Gita*, "Salutations to thee, O Vyasa [the incarnation of Krishna who compiled the essential Vedic literature. Thou art of mighty intellect, and thine eyes are as large as a full-blown lotus. It was thou who brightened this lamp of wisdom, filling it with the oil of the *Mahabharata*." Shankara also readily points out that it is Bhagavan Krishna "whose glories are sung by the verses of the *Vedas*, of whom the singers of the *Sama* sing, and of whose glories the *Upanishads* proclaim in full choir." This would seem to indicate that Shankara was encouraging everyone to read *Bhagavad Gita* and *Mahabharata* as written by Srila Vyasadeva to understand the conclusion of spiritual knowledge.

This would also give evidence that Shankara's own personal beliefs were different from the philosophy that he taught. There is no evidence that makes this clearer than texts eight and nine of his *Meditations on the Bhagavad Gita* as follows:

> I offer my respectful obeisances unto the supreme personality of Godhead, Krishna, the transcendental, blissful husband of the Goddess of Fortune, whose mercy turns the dumb into eloquent speakers and enables the lame to cross mountains. Let all obeisances be unto the Supreme Lord Sri Krishna, whom Brahma, Varuna, Indra, Rudra, the Maruts, and all divine beings praise with the divine hymns of the Vedas and their supplementary parts, such as the Upanishads, whom the followers of the Sama Veda glorify with song, whom great mystics see with their minds absorbed in perfect meditation and of whom all the hosts of demigods and demons know not the limitations. To him, the Supreme Lord, let there be all obeisance.

Near the end of his life, Shankara wrote his *Bhaja Govindam* prayers. Verses 1 and 34, which are the conclusive verses in these prayers, are often overlooked by his followers. Yet they were written especially for those who might miss the actual purport of the *Vedas*. He wrote in verse one, "Worship Govinda [another name of Krishna], worship Govinda, worship Govinda, you intellectual fools. At the end of your life all your grammatical arguments will not help you." And again in verse 34 he writes, "Worship Govinda, worship Govinda, worship Govinda, Oh fool. Other than chanting the Lord's names, there is no other way to cross the material ocean [of birth and death]." In the final book that Shankaracharya wrote, the *Prabodh Sudhakar*, he established his true philosophy. He pointed out that God has two eternal forms, which are both personal and impersonal, that latter of which is difficult to realize. The supreme form is the beautiful and divine Lord Krishna, who appeared on this earth in the Yadu dynasty. *Without devotion to Lord Krishna, one's heart cannot be fully purified.* Thus, as he says, it is one's own ill fortune if one is not attracted to the form and pastimes of Lord Krishna. In this way, even Shankaracharya emphasized that it is Krishna who is the Supreme form of God, and that the supreme form of God realization is through the process of worshiping him and chanting Krishna's holy names, which is the sure way of liberation from material existence. Ramanuja (AD 1017-1137) did not accept Shankara's Mayavada interpretation of the *Vedanta sutras* and sought to expose Shankara's contradictory arguments which were actually in defiance of the real Vedic conclusions. He felt there was little difference between Shakara's philosophy and the Buddhists. Ramanuja wrote over forty books, but the three major commentaries for which Ramanuja is most known is his *Vedanta Sangraha*, which is on the *Vedas*; the *Sri Bhasya* on the *Vedanta sutras*; and *Bhagavad Gita Bhasya*, which is on *Bhagavad Gita*. His prominent theme is his opposition to impersonal monism, especially of Shankara, and the support of Vaishnavism, worship of the one god Vishnu or Bhagavan Sri Krishna.

Ramanuja's interpretation of Vedanta, as related in his *Sri Bhasya* commentary, establishes that God is one and the soul is a part of God, but that it remains individual in nature even after liberation from the body, rather than merging into the Absolute. This is called *vishishthadvaita*. He also explains that the process for liberation includes surrendering to the personal form of God. Ramanuja accepted that the Supreme and the individual living entities are one in spiritual quality, but the individual souls are very small and God is unlimited, and between them is a relationship based on *bhakti*, or spiritual love. By logical reasoning, he taught that just as the *jiva* controls his own body and uses it as an instrument, God controls the whole material creation as well as the *jiva* souls within. The soul is eternal and after being liberated from material entanglement lives in an eternal spiritual body. The soul is the eternal servant of God, in which case the soul becomes fully happy after meeting and engaging in service to God. This, therefore, is the goal of the Vedic spiritual process. Madhvacharya (AD 1239-1319) was another prominent philosopher who wrote a commentary on the *Vedanta sutra* and the *Gita*, along with more than thirty other books. He was also a Vaishnava who worked to combat Shankara's impersonal philosophy. Madhava accepted the renounced order of *sannyasa* when he was only eleven years old. He studied the Vedanta, and after traveling to the Himalayas, he met Vyasadeva, who still lives in the mountains and who taught him to teach the glories of Vaishnava *bhakti*. Thereafter, he traveled around the country and established the importance of *bhakti* through his talent of debating with scriptural evidence. Madhva's interpretation of Vedanta, as found in his *Tatparya Nirnayas*, also presents Vedanta philosophy as dualistic (*dvaita*), similar to Ramanuja's, but more developed.

Madhva taught pure dualism and that there are three energies: spiritual, marginal, and inferior. The Lord is of the superior spiritual energy and controller of all other energies. The living entities are the marginal energy since they can be engrossed spiritually or materially. And the material energy is inferior due to its temporary nature. The Lord and the living entities are eternal and always distinct, but the Lord is always completely transcendental to the material world. The Lord is the ultimate cause of the creation, maintenance, and annihilation of the material manifestation, thereby being completely independent while the living entities are completely dependent on the Lord. They remain bound up in material energy by the result of their own *karma* or activities based on their fruitive desires. But Madhva pointed out that through *bhakti*, devotion to God, people could eliminate their *karma* and reawaken their real spiritual identity and return to their natural position in the spiritual world. Nimbarka also delivered a commentary called *Vedanta Parijata Saurabh* based on the dualistic idea. He was born in South India, somewhere near the Godavari River, but it is not known exactly when. The tradition is that he was initiated by Narada Muni, another eternally living sage. In his commentary, he establishes that God is one with but separate from each soul. This is called the *dvaitadvaitvad* philosophy.

This means that God and the individual souls are spiritual in quality, yet God is infinite, and the living entities are infinitesimal. Nimbarka also explained that Radha Krishna are the ultimate form of God, and the basis of the topmost spiritual development is devotion to RadhaKrishna. Vallabhacharya (1478-1530) also wrote a commentary on the *Vedanta sutras*, called the *Anu Bhashya*. He also wrote on the *Bhagavatam*, along with a few other books, which emphasized that the *Bhagavatam* is the essence of all spiritual and devotional knowledge. His philosophy is called *shuddhadvaita vad*, or pure monism. This established that Krishna was the supreme form of God, and that the soul is not merely a part of God's energy, but is qualitatively the same as God, but small in potency. Furthermore, Krishna gives a person everything for spiritual development when one surrenders with love to him. This knowledge is said to have started from Lord Shiva (Rudra), and came down to Vishnuswami, then Gyanadeva, Nath Dev, and on down to Vallabhacharya. This is why it is also called the Ru-dra *sampradaya* or disciplic succession. Vallabhacharya was born in Raipur. By the time he was eleven years old he went to Kashi to study under Madhavendra Puri and became well educated in the knowledge of the Vedic scripture. After staying for a time in Vrindavana, he traveled to the major holy places of India and spread the understanding of devotion to Lord Krishna. After he returned to Vrindavana he started the temple of Sri Nathji at Govardhan. He established a structured form of deity worship centered around the deity of Lord Krishna. When he was twenty-eight, he was married and had two sons, Gopinatha and Vitthalanath. Vitthal became known as Goswamiji and started six more temples, of which four are in the area of Vrindavana, two in Kamban and one in Gokul. Kashi was the home to Vallabhacharya the last years of his life. It is said that once during bathing in the river, in front of hundreds of people, a big bright light appeared near him and he ascended up into the sky and disappeared into the spiritual world. Sri Chaitanya Mahaprabhu (AD 1486-1534) also strongly opposed Shankara's Mayavada philosophy and established the principle of *achintya bhedabheda tattva*. This specified that the Supreme and the individual soul are inconceivably and simultaneously one and different. This means that the Supreme and the *jiva* souls are the same in quality, being eternally spiritual, but always separate individually. The *jivas* are small and subject to being influenced by the material energy, while the Supreme is infinite and always above and beyond the material manifestation. Sri Chaitanya taught that the direct meaning of the Vedic *shastras* is that the living entities are to engage in devotional service, *bhakti*, to the Supreme, Bhagavan Sri Krishna. Through this practice, there can develop a level of communication between God and the individual by which God will lovingly reveal himself to those who become qualified. In this understanding, the Vedic theistic philosophy of Vaishnavism reached its climax. Sri Chaitanya Mahaprabhu, who is considered and was established by Vedic scripture as the most recent incarnation of God, did not become much involved in writing. In fact, he only wrote eight verses called the *Shikshastaka*, but his followers compiled extensive Sanskrit literature that documented his life and fully explained his teachings. However, it is one of his followers, Baladeva Vidyabushana, who wrote a commentary on the *Vedanta sutras* called *Govindabhasya*. Baladeva Vidyabushana also wrote a very important commentary on the Vedanta called *Sri Bhasya*, and established the individual nature of the soul. Baladeva had met Pandit Sri Radha Damodara, a disciple of Sri Rasikananda Deva, who was a great follower of *Sri Chaitanya Mahaprabhu*. Sri Radha Damodar instructed Baladeva in the pastimes and teachings of Sri Chaitanya and the Vaishnava Gaudiya tradition. Later Baladeva went to Vrindavana to stay with Vishvanatha Chakravarti Thakur to continue his progress. One day in the royal court in Jaipur, the Ramanuja pandits were arguing that the Gaudiya line did not have any written commentary on the Vedanta. In other words, without a written commentary, they were not viewed as authorized. So the Ramanuja Pandits said the Gaudiya Vaishnavas should simply join them since they were an authorized line with their own written commentary. The Jaipur king, who was also a follower of the Gaudiya line, sent word of this to Vishvanatha Chakravarti Thakur asking that if there was a commentary it should be sent at once. Sri Vishvanatha was too old and infirm to go, so he sent Baladeva to Jaipur. Baladeva was an excellent scholar and challenged the Ramanuja pandits in the huge assembly. Even after much debate, none of them could stand before Baladeva's conclusions. However, he said that the Gaudiya Vaishnava line or *sampradaya* did not write a commentary on the *Vedanta sutras* because they accepted Vyasadeva's *Srimad Bhagavatam* as the final commentary on Vedanta. The Ramanuja pandits could not accept this. So Baladeva promised to show a commentary to them in a few days. Baladeva, in a troubled state, then went to the temple to pray to Rupa Gosvami's deity, Lord Govinda, and related everything that had happened to the deity, who is still one of the prominent deities in Jaipur today. That night Baladeva had a dream in which Sri Govinda told him to write the commentary and it would be perfect. Thereafter, he meditated on the lotus feet of the deity of Govinda and wrote the powerful commentary and called it *Govindabhasya,* signifying that it was the words of Sri Krishna himself. He arrived at the assembly hall of the king and presented the commentary to the Ramanuja pandits, who were speechless. The Gaudiya tradition was declared victorious and that is when the pandits gave Baladeva the name of Vidyabhushana, meaning one whose decoration is knowledge. The Ramanuja pandits also accepted Baladeva as their acharya and desired to become his disciples. However, with humility he said that the Ramanuja or Shri *sampradaya* was also one of the four prominent spiritual successions. Baladeva wrote a number of other books besides the *Govindabhasya*, among the most noted are *Siddhantadarpana*, *Vedantasa mantaka*, and *Prameya Ratnavali*. All of these presented different levels of spiritual understanding based on the fact that the Vedic knowledge is the best to use for realizing the supreme lord Sri Krishna and the ultimate form of reality.

There is, of course, one more commentary on the *Vedanta sutras* that we cannot neglect. Srila Vyasadeva, the original author of the *Vedanta sutras*, was still not satisfied after writing it. After explaining this perplexing situation to his spiritual master, Narada Muni, he was advised to write the *Srimad Bhagavatam* (also called the *Bhagavata Purana*). After doing so, Vyasadeva considered it his own commentary on the *Vedanta sutras* and the complete explanation and conclusion of all Vedic philosophy. This is why, Sri Chaitanya never cared for writing a commentary on the Vedanta sutras, because he considered Srimad Bhagavatam to be the topmost commentary that had already been written, which will be discussed soon. This *Srimad Bhagavatam* is part of the Vedic literature called the *Itihasas*.

The *Itihasas*, or supplementary Vedic literature, helps explain the rituals of the *Vedas* and the highly compressed philosophy of the *Vedanta sutras* by using historical events of the universe and factual stories of many great sages, demigods, and so forth. Included in the *Itihasas* is the *Mahabharata*, written by Srila Vyasadeva. It is an historical epic about the great kingdom of *Bharatavarsa*, or the region of India. It contains 110,000 couplets making it the longest poem and greatest epic in world literature. It is divided into eighteen sections called *parvas*, such as the *Adi Parva*, etc. It is a treasure house of Indian lore and holds within it a code of life for ethical, social and spiritual relations. Throughout this great epic every sort of human situation is described and every kind of emotion is aroused.

There is a saying that if it is not in the *Mahabharata* then it is not to be found. The *Mahabharata* deals with the activities of the Pandavas and Krishna's relations, as well as topics that include the creation of the world, history of the sages, *dharma*, politics, military strategies, proper behavior of a king, and ways of spirituality and devotion to God. It includes the essence of the *Upanishads* and Vedic teachings, and the famous *Bhagavad Gita*. The *Mahabharata* also explains a great variety of historical incidents, mainly consisting of the story of how the demoniac Kuru dynasty cheated the family of pious Pandavas, time and time again out of their rightful heritage of the kingdom of northern India. Finally, after the Pandavas are exiled to the forest and attempted peaceful means to gain their right to the throne, the epic centers around the eighteen day battle at Kuruksetra, a place which is still found in Madhyadesa, a three-hour train ride north of Delhi. There the Pandava army defeated the Kurus and their soldiers. This is also where Sri Krishna speaks the *Bhagavad Gita* to his friend Arjuna just before the battle takes place. The *Bhagavad Gita* is from chapters 25 to 42 of the *Bishmaparva* section of the *Ma-habharata*. It is a classic of Indian literature and considered the essence of all Vedic knowledge. It is the indispensable *Upanishad* and the important handbook or guide for traveling the spiritual path to God realization. It is especially good for those who do not have much time for reading or who cannot go very deeply into studying the Vedic literature. It contains knowledge of the soul, law of karma, reincarnation, attaining the Supreme, knowledge of God, and the essential purpose of life. It ultimately reveals the supremacy of the path of devotion, bhakti yoga, as the best means for regaining our awareness of our relationship with the Supreme Lord. More importantly, the *Bhagavad Gita* is the direct instruction from God to his devotee. The *Mahabharata* is especially meant to draw the attention of people to the *Bhagavad Gita* through the format of an exciting, historical adventure, which is certainly found in the *Mahabharata*. The *Ramayana* is a similar epic, consisting of twenty-four thousand verses, and first written during the time of Lord Ramachandra by the great poet Valmiki, which describes the life of Lord Ramachandra, an incarnation of God, and his wife, Sita. This is also a most touching and exciting adventure which explains how Lord Ramachandra lived in the forest and fought against and killed the great demon Ravana and his armies in order to rescue his wife, Sita, who had been kidnapped. Many other stories are included in this storehouse of wisdom that has been an inspiration for thousands of years to all people who have read it. In the incarnation of Lord Ramachandra, God appears as the perfect king and ruler, and inspires all his subjects with the greatest love for him. Even though the *Itihasas* are accepted as supplementary Vedic literature, the *acharyas* such as Shankara, Ramanuja, and Madhva have all presented the *Itihasas* as valid Vedic evidence and wrote commentaries on *Bhagavad Gita*. Actually Shankara thought the *Gita* was in fact the epitome of the essentials of all Vedic teaching. Madhva, commenting on the *Vedanta sutras* (2.1.6), quotes the *Bhavisya Purana*, which states, "The *Rig-Veda, Yajurveda, Samaveda, Atharvaveda, Mahabharata, Pancaratra*, and the original *Ramayana* are all considered Vedic literature. The Vaishnava supplements, the *Puranas*, are also Vedic literature." The *Chandogya Upanisad* (7.1.4) mentions the *Puranas* and *Itihasas* as the fifth *Veda*. The *Srimad Bhagavatam* (1.4.20) also states, "The four divisions of the original sources of knowledge [the *Vedas*] were made separately. But the historical facts and authentic stories mentioned in the *Puranas* are called the fifth *Veda*." Therefore, the Vedas themselves not only accept the four Vedas, the Upanishads, and Vedanta sutras, but also the Mahabharata, Bhagavad Gita, the Ramayana, and the Puranas as being authentic Vedic literature.

The point is, to be accepted as Vedic literature it must present the same purpose as the original texts. But if it deviates from the Vedic conclusion or is a hodgepodge of various concocted philosophies, as are many viewpoints that one will find merged under the name of "Hinduism," then it cannot be relied upon. Therefore, to be sure something is authorized, we only accept the established Vedic teachings that are supported in the many Vedic texts. So Buddhism, Jainism and Sikhism, which do not refer to or support the conclusions of the Vedic texts, are considered non-Vedic, although outgrowths of Vedic philosophy and accepted as part of Hinduism by some.

Another important part of the *Itihasas* is the *Puranas*. The *Puranas* are the histories of the universe and contain many stories that *took place on earth or even on other planets* and dimensions, or in which superhuman powers are commonplace. As we pointed out earlier, Vedic knowledge often consists of information about things from beyond our own sense perception or experience. We can be assured of its authenticity because of the fact that many Vedic scholars such as Sukadeva, Maitreya, Madhva, Ramanuja, and others have reached *spiritual perfection with the help of information found in the Puranas*. Each *Purana* is supposed to contain five basic subjects and in some cases ten. These include: (1) the creation of the world, (2) its destruction and recreation, (3) the genealogy of the patriarchs and the demigods, (4) the reigns of the Manus (who are the *avataras* in each duration of time known as a *manvantara*), (5) and the history of the Solar and Lunar dynasties. Many of them also include descriptions of the activities of the incarnations of God, as well as the great sages and devotees of God. One thing that may seem somewhat confusing is that the stories are not in any particular chronological order and may be related at any time according to need. This is primarily due to the fact that the *Puranas* are generally related in a dialogue of questions and answers between sages and saints, or masters and disciples. Then the histories and stories are related in the answers. Other subjects included in various *Puranas* are geography, astrology, use of military weapons, organization of society, duties of different classes of men, characteristics of social leaders, predictions of the future, law of reincarnation and *karma*, analysis of the material elements, symptoms of consciousness, how the illusory energy works, the practice of yoga, meditation, spiritual experiences, realizations of the Absolute, etc. The *Puranas* explain more clearly and completely the spiritual philosophy found in the four original *Veda samhitas*. Thus, they especially are meant for all classes of people. Since all men are not on the same level of consciousness and are spread over many different types of thinking, feeling and desiring, the *Puranas* are divided so that any class of people can take advantage of them and utilize them to get out of the material entanglement either gradually or rapidly. So depending on their position in life, people may use the particular *Puranas* that are most suited for them.

The *Puranas* are divided into two main groups consisting of the primary *MahaPuranas* and the secondary *UpaPuranas*. The *UpaPuranas* consist of eighteen, entitled: *Sanatkumara, Narasimha, Naradiya, Shiva, Durvasasa, Kapila, Manava, Ausanasa, Varuna, Kalika, Samba, Nandi, Saura, Parasara, Aditya, Mahesvara, Bhagavata* or *Bhargava*, and *Vasistha*. The eighteen *MahaPuranas* are divided into three groups. One group considered to be related to the mode of *tamoguna*, or the lower nature, consists of the *Linga, Skanda, Agni, Matsya, Kurma,* and *Shiva* (or sometimes the *Vayu*) *Puranas*. These are usually related to Lord Shiva. The next group is usually related to Lord Brahma and is considered connected with *rajaguna*, the mode of action or passion. These consist of the *Brahma, Brahmanda, Brahma Vaivarta, Markandeya, Bhavisya,* and *Vamana Puranas*. The third group relates to Lord Vishnu with *satoguna* prevailing, which is the mode of purity or goodness. These are the *Vishnu, Bhagavata, Narada* or *Naradiya, Garuda, Padma,* and *Varaha Puranas*.

This review of the *Puranas* will exhibit some of the many topics found in each one. So that we can get an understanding of the basic content of each *Purana* and see the direction in awareness and understanding that can be reached by the study of particular *Puranas*. The *Linga Purana* has about eleven thousand verses in two sections. It focuses mainly on the glories and activities of Lord Shiva. *This Purana includes the manifestation of the Shivalinga and its worship, the worship and fasting days for Shiva, descriptions of the holy city of Kashi (Varanasi), Shiva's thousand names, his marriage to Parvati,* the appearance of Ganesh, and more. The later section also includes some descriptions of the glories of Lord Vishnu and some of his pastimes, as well as more about the worship of Lord Shiva. The *Skanda Purana* is the largest with around eighty-one thousand verses. It is divided into seven sections, mostly about Lord Vishnu and Shiva. It covers many different topics, some of which include the holiness of places like Kedar, Badarikashrama, Mathura, Kashi, Dwarka, and many other places and sacred rivers. It also covers worship of Shiva, the austerities of Parvati, worship of Vishnu and stories of prominent devotees, as well as activities and worship of Lord Rama. The *Agni Purana* has about fifteen thousand verses. Herein Agni, the fire god, explains to the sage Vashishtha many spiritual instructions. These include descriptions of the Lord's incarnations, the universal creation, the greatness of the Ganges River, the science of astrology, religious disciplines, yoga practice, Ayurveda, knowledge of Brahman, and the art of *bhakti*, or devotional service. The *Matsya Purana* has about fourteen thousand verses, which begins with the conversation between Lord Matsya and Manu. Again, it includes many topics, among which you can find descriptions of the universal creation, the family and descendants of King Iksvaku, Surya and Chandra, along with the ten avataras of God. It also relates the principles of worship and fasting on holy days, the pastimes of Parvati and Shiva, their marriage, and other stories.

The KurmaPurana has around seventeen thousand verses about the occurrences of the day of Brahma called *LakshmiKalpa*. Herein, the Lord's incarnation as Kurma presents his teachings to the great sages. These include the manifestation and maintenance of the universe, the pastimes of Lord Krishna, the greatness of Kashi and other holy places, the effects of devotion (*bhakti*) to God that everyone should strive to attain, and the duties or *dharma* for liberation. The, Vayu Purana or sometimes the *Shiva Purana*, has about twenty-four thousand verses. In this book Vayu, the wind god, describes events of the present *kalpa*, or day of Brahma. It contains the usual information that a *Purana* explains, such as the process of creation, the incarnations of God, the *manvantaras*, the glories of the Narmada River, and detailed accounts of Lord Shiva. The *Brahma Purana* has around ten thousand verses. This includes the stories of Lord Ramachandra, many stories of Lord Krishna, along with those of Surya the sun god, and the birth of Parvati and her marriage to Shiva, and other aspects of the Vedic sciences. The *Brahmananda Purana* has around twelve thousand verses in four parts. This provides descriptions of future *kalpas* (days of Brahma). Included are descriptions of the holy place of Naimisharanya, Bharatvarsha (the area of India) and other places in the world. It also describes other planetary systems, Svayambhuva Manu and other *manvantaras*, the activities of Lord Krishna, and the dynasties of King Iksvaku, Yadu and Vrishni, along with the dynasties and characteristics of people in the age of Kali Yuga. There are also descriptions of the creation and annihilation of the universe.

The *Brahma Vaivarta Purana* has about eighteen thousand verses in four sections. This *Purana* is known for the information it provides about Lord Vishnu and Shiva, and shows their unity. It also includes the basic topics of most *Puranas*, such as the account of the universal creation. It also provides 129 chapters of many stories of the pastimes of Radha and Krishna and how to worship him. It also discusses Goloka, the divinity of Krishna and appearance of Radha, and numerous descriptions of her, the birth and marriage of Tulasi, the story of Vrinda, and more. There are also accounts of Narada going to Shiva's abode and receiving instructions, along with activities of Ganesh, Kartikeya, Parashurama, and others. The *Markandeya Purana* has about nine thousand verses. Here we find the conversation between the sages Markandeya and Jaimini. A wide range of topics are discussed, a few of which include Lord Balarama's pilgrimage when he refused to take part in the war of Kurukshetra, stories of Draupadi's five sons, Dattatreya, the lineage of Vaivasvata Manu, stories of Lord Rama, Krishna, his incarnations, and various spiritual instructions. The *Bhavishya Purana* has about fourteen thousand verses in five sections, or *parvas*. This deals with the characteristics of Brahma, *dharma*, worship of Vishnu and Shiva for worldly prosperity as well as liberation, and information about Surya. There are also instructions for religious discipline, charity, etc. The fifth section is what this *Purana* is most known for, which contains the descriptions of the kings and characteristics of the future of this age of Kali Yuga. However, there are now parts of this *Purana*, namely of the fifth section, that are completely lost. Furthermore, some scholars feel that certain portions of it, such as the *Uttara Parva*, were later additions that were separate from the original. So though many people look to the *Bhavishya Purana* for its predictions of the future, it is not considered fully dependable because of the additions and deletions. However, numerous predictions of the future are also found in other *Puranas*, many of which can help substantiate those in the *Bhavishya* by comparisons.

The *Vamana Purana* has about ten thousand verses and describes the occurrences that take place in the day of Brahma called the *KurmaKalpa*. It relates the fighting between the demons and demigods, Daksha's unfortunate sacrificial ritual, the activities of Goddess Durga and Parvati, the greatness of Vishnu, and the conversation between Prahlada and King Bali, as well as the activities of Lord Krishna and his devotees.

The *Varaha Purana* has about twenty-four thousand verses. Herein there is a conversation between Lord Varaha and Bhumidevi (the earth goddess) about the manifestation of Gauri (Parvati) and her sons Ganesh and Kartikeya. Gauri's battle with the demon Mahishasura, and the greatness of holy sites like Mathura and other places are also described. It also has more about general Vedic philosophy. The *Narada Purana* has around twenty-five thousand verses. This *Purana* includes the teachings of the four Kumaras who offer their advice regarding such things as duties in family life and religious practice. There are also descriptions of the appearance and activities of Shukadeva Gosvami who learned the knowledge of the *Bhagavatam* and recited it for King Pariksit, along with the pastimes and characteristics of Lord Vishnu, Surya, Ganesh, Shiva, Durga, and others. It also offers descriptions of the other *Puranas*, as well as the greatness of such holy places as Haridwar, Kashi, Kuruksetra, Mathura, Vrindavana, and other places.

The *Garuda Purana* has around nineteen thousand verses in which Lord Vishnu answers questions of his carrier, Garuda, on Vedic topics and activities of the day of Brahma called the *Tark-shyaKalpa*. This *Purana* primarily relates the glories of Lord Vishnu. It contains the thousand names of Vishnu (the Vishnu Sahasranama), ways of meditating on Lord Vishnu and worship of Lord Krishna. It also includes the pastimes of Lord Rama, the process of yoga, types of charity, Sankhya philosophy, descriptions of the spiritual domain, the celestial regions, and the process for attaining liberation from material existence.

The *Padma Purana* is a large book of fifty-five thousand verses in five sections. It includes the important stories of Lord Krishna and Vrindavana, Lord Rama, and other stories on the importance of various holy places, such as Pushkar, Jagannatha Puri, Kashi (Varanasi), Prayag (Allahabad), Gaya, and the Narmada and Ganga rivers. It also includes a section called the *Bhagavata Mahatmya* on the glories and greatness of the *Bhagavata Purana*. The *Devi Bhagavat* is another prominent *Purana* not mentioned in the main groups that is said to be written by Srila Vyasadeva. It has eighteen verses in twelve cantos. It offers descriptions of the other eighteen *Puranas* and the eighteen

Upa Puranas. It also describes the twenty-eight Vyasadevas who appeared at the end of each of the twenty-eight Dvaparayugas during the present time period known as the *manvantara* of Svayambhuva Manu. It also contains the typical information found in most *Puranas*, but the tenth canto specializes in information about the goddesses Maha Kali, Maha Lakshmi and Maha Sarasvati. The ninth canto explains that Vishnu and Shiva ultimately appeared from Lord Krishna, and both Lakshmi and Sarasvati manifested from the Supreme Goddess Srimati Radharani, while Durga appeared in front of both Radha and Krishna. This shows that Radha and Krishna are the source of all other forms of the Divine. The *Devi Bhagavat Purana* says, as do other *Puranas*, that Vyasadeva appears at the end of every Dvaparayuga to compile and write the four *Vedas*, and to reorganize the *Puranas* for the good of the people of Kali Yuga. *This means that this information is eternal and is the same as that produced in its written form in the earliest Kali Yuga* many thousands of years ago. Out of all the *Puranas*, many scholars seem to agree that the *Vishnu Purana* seems to conform most closely to what a *Purana* is expected to be. It has around twenty-three thousand verses. It contains the five essential subjects that a *Purana* is supposed to relate and also describes many other topics that are dealt with in detail. The central theme is praise of Vishnu, so it describes many aspects of him and prominent stories of the Lord's famous devotees, such as Prahlada, Dhruva, Prithu, and others. It also contains many stories of Lord Krishna in Vrindavana and Mathura, and his incarnations, along with the evils and predictions of the age of Kali Yuga, and many other facets of Vedic knowledge.

This *Purana* is quite similar to the contents of the *Bhagavata Purana*, otherwise called *Srimad Bhagavatam*, which is also centered around the theme of praise of Lord Krishna, the source of all other incarnations of God, and relates many stories of Lord Krishna's pastimes.

The Bhagavatam, or Bhagavata Purana, is held to be the most significant of all the Puranas. It has about eighteen thousand verses in twelve cantos and is the most widely read and one of the greatest works of devotion ever written. It is a book that goes to the core of understanding God and reveals the bliss of devotion to the Supreme Being, the depths of which make the other Vedic gods, such as Shiva, also hanker for it. This *Purana* describes how Vyasadeva came to write it and details the pastimes of the various *avataras* of God and his prominent devotees, but especially the pastimes of Lord Krishna. Other descriptions include the process of the universal creation and annihilation, the characteristics of the four ages or *yugas*, and much in the way of the teachings of Lord Krishna and Vedic knowledge. Five hundred years ago Sri Chaitanya Mahaprahu, along with other scholars of the *Vedas*, relied on and researched the *Bhagavatam* extensively for information on the Absolute Truth and became immersed in many stories about Sri Krishna in their spiritual ecstasies. The *Bhagavatam* is Sri Vyasadeva's own commentary on all the Vedanta philosophy. It brings to light all the different aspects of the Absolute Truth, but especially the personal characteristics of Bhagavan Sri Krishna as the final conclusion of all Vedic understanding. This is why those who are impersonalists or monists, believing God ultimately has no form and therefore performs no activities, never reach the *Bhagavatam* in their Vedic studies. But if they do read the *Bhagavatam*, they are sure to interpret it in an impersonalistic way and thus deprive themselves of the truth and purity that they could derive from it. *Srimad Bhagavatam* is considered the postgraduate study of the *Bhagavad Gita*. The *Bhagavatam* does not elaborate on worship of the other demigods or on rituals that award various temporary material benedictions as do some of the other *Vedas* and *Puranas*. Therefore, the *Bhagavatam* completely transcends all other philosophical viewpoints of the Vedic literature. This is confirmed in the *Garuda Purana* (*Brahma Kanda*, 1.45) where it states: "The wise declare knowledge to be manifold, consisting of various grades: high, low, and middle. All that knowledge is found in the *Bhagavata Purana*. Hence, *Bhagavata* is the highest of all *Puranas*." Furthermore, in the "*artho yam brahmasutranam* "verse, it fully states: "The *Srimad Bhagavatam* is the authorized explanation of *Brahmasutra*, and it is a further explanation of *Mahabharata*. It is the expansion of the *Gayatri* mantra and the essence of all Vedic knowledge. This *Srimad Bhagavatam*, containing eighteen thousand verses, is known as the explanation of all Vedic literature." It is explained in the first verse of the *Bhagavatam* that it aims only at selfless devotional service to Lord Krishna. This is what separates it from all other *Puranas*. It ultimately delivers one to the Divine bliss found in the loving pastimes that Lord Krishna displays in his spiritual abode of Goloka Vrindavana. This topic is beyond the *Vedas* and *Upanishads*, which do not go near to that depth or level of spiritual understanding. The s*hruti* scripture (*Vedas, Brahmanas, Upanishads*), besides giving information on the process of rituals, primarily consists of knowledge of the futility of material existence, the temporary nature of the material creation, the bondage of the *jiva* souls in this existence, and the spiritual nature of the individual souls and the Supreme Being.

They explain that the goal of life is liberation from the material worlds by returning back to the spiritual domain through the process of understanding *karma*, spiritual knowledge, renunciation, and devotion (*bhakti*). They do not explain much beyond this, or at least the finer details of what is beyond. They do not take you to the bliss of spiritual activities, nor the pastimes of *Goloka Vrindavana, the most intimate and confidential spiritual abode of the Lord.* That is why it is especially the *Bhagavatam* that begins to explain the supreme bliss of devotional love in the eternal pastimes that go on in the *Vaikuntha planets*, and in the Vrindavana atmosphere. It is this *Bhagavata Purana* that first reveals the supremacy of Lord Krishna's love and the reciprocation that he provides above all other forms of God. The *Bhagavatam* is the *highest manifestation of the bliss that comes from purely concentrating on the Supreme* without any material inebriates. It is from this platform that one can go deeper and deeper into such love and bliss, which then manifests even profounder realizations and experiences. The second verse of the *Srimad Bhagavatam* explains this point and what this *Purana* consists of and who can understand it: Completely rejecting all religious activities which are materially motivated, the *Bhagavata Purana* propounds the highest truth, which is understandable by those devotees who are fully pure in heart. The highest truth is reality distinguished from illusion for the welfare of all. Such truth uproots the threefold miseries. This beautiful *Bhagavatam*, compiled by the great sage Vyasadeva, is sufficient in itself for God realization. What is the need for any other scripture? As soon as one attentively and submissively hears the message of *Bhagavatam*, by this culture of knowledge the Supreme Lord is established within the heart. As it is stated, this knowledge can be understood by those who are pure in heart. This means that those who are envious, atheists, or who read it with some ulterior motive will never be able to fully comprehend it. But for those who listen submissively and sincerely with an open mind, all the mysteries of the highest truth will gradually be revealed. Let us help unveil that reality in our souls, practicing the vedas, having more *somic states* in our lives, experiencing that reality in "drops." That highest truth is "reality distinguished from illusion for the welfare of all." Not that we can make up our own reality, but we must understand what is actually reality.

Even though we can find information about Lord Krishna's pastimes in all the *Puranas*, particularly the *Skanda Purana*, *Padma Purana*, *Vishnu Purana*, and the 129 chapters of the *Brahmavaivarta Purana*, as well as details about Radharani in the *Devi Bhagavat*, there is a difference in the *Bhagavatam*. The difference is that the other texts relate the pastimes like a reporter giving a description of the events. But in the *Bhagavatam*, especially in the tenth canto, the *bliss* of these pastimes is presented from a participant's point of view, one who is involved, and not from a spectator who is merely watching and describing the proceedings. This is the way Vyasadeva was inspired by Narada, and how the *Bhagavatam* had been spoken by Shukadeva Gosvami to King Pariksit. King Pariksit had seven days left to live and asked for the most essential spiritual truth, so Shukadeva Gosvami spoke the *Bhagavatam* to him. This is also how the reader can dive deep into the *rasa*, or the taste of the loving relationship that is displayed between Lord Krishna and his devotees in Goloka Vrindavana. This loving bliss is not experienced or seen in the relationships with Shiva, Durga, Brahma, or Vishnu, or in their abodes. It is only available with Sri Krishna in Vrindavana. It is this bliss, this ever increasing happiness, for which we are always searching, intentionally or not, knowingly or unknowingly. This is what the *Bhagavatam* delivers for one who can dive deep enough. Many *quotations regarding the extraordinary importance of the Bhagavatam* can be found in several other *Puranas*, such as the *Bhagavata Mahatmya* section of the *Padma Purana*, wherein we find such verses as the following: The holy scripture known as *Srimad Bhagavatam* was expounded in this age of Kali by the *sage Sukadeva Gosvami [Vyasadeva's son]* with the object of completely destroying the fear of being caught in the jaws of the serpent of time. There is no means other than this conducive to the purification of the mind. One gets to hear *Srimad Bhagavatam* only when there is virtue earned in one's past lives (1.1112). All the evils of Kali Yuga [this present age of quarrel and confusion] will surely disappear at the very chanting of *Srimad Bhagavatam*, even as wolves take flight at the very roar of a lion (1.62) ... If you seek the highest destiny, read even yourself daily one half of a quarter of a verse of *Srimad Bhagavatam* (3.33) ... Indeed, this is the righteous course prescribed in the Kali age for washing away all agony, poverty, misfortune and sin as well as for the conquest of passion and anger. Otherwise the illusory energy of the Lord is most difficult to get rid of even for the gods. How then can it be set aside by men? Hence, the course of hearing *Srimad Bhagavatam* has been recommended (3.6465) ... Like bubbles appearing in water or mosquitoes among living beings, *those who remain deprived of hearing an exposition of Srimad Bhagavatam are born only to die (5.63)*. There are many other verses in the *Padma Purana* that point out the potency and importance of the *Bhagavatam*.

The importance of the book is also described in the *Bhagavatam* itself: This *Bhagavata Purana* is as brilliant as the sun, and it has arisen just after the departure of Lord Krishna to his own abode accompanied by religion, knowledge, etc. *Persons who have lost their vision due to the dense darkness of ignorance in the age of Kali shall get light from this Purana* (Bhag.1.3.43). Another example (*Bhag.*12.13.1416) is where Suta Gosvami emphasizes its significance, stating that the glorious *Bhagavatam* is considered to be the cream of all the *Upanishads*, and a man who is satisfied with tasting the nectar from it will not find such pleasure anywhere else. "All other Puranic scriptures shine forth in the assembly of saintly devotees only as long as that great ocean of nectar, *Srimad Bhagavatam*, is not heard. *Srimad Bhagavatam* is declared to be the essence of all Vedanta philosophy. One who has felt satisfaction from its nectarean mellow will never be attracted to any other literature. Just as the Ganga is the greatest of all rivers, Lord Achyuta, the supreme among deities and Lord Shambhu [Shiva], the greatest of Vaishnavas, so *Srimad Bhagavatam* is the greatest of all *Puranas.*" Suta Gosvami also says (*Bhag.*1.2.3), Let me offer my respectful obeisances unto him [Sukadeva], the spiritual master of all sages, the son of Vyasadeva, who, out of his great compassion for those gross materialists.

Who struggle to cross over the darkest regions of material existence, spoke this most confidential supplement to the cream of Vedic knowledge, after having personally assimilated it by experience. Srila Suta Goswami explains the benefit of studying the *Bhagavatam* in this way, "Simply by giving aural reception to this Vedic literature, the feeling for loving devotional service to Lord Krishna, the supreme personality of Godhead, sprouts up at once to extinguish the fire of lamentation, illusion and fearfulness." (*Bhag.*1.7.7) When Maharaja Pariksit learned that he had merely seven more days to live, only a week to bring his life to any kind of spiritual perfection, he asked the great sage Sukadeva Gosvami what he should do. Shukadeva was the son of Srila Vyasadeva, the compiler of the Vedic literature. At the time, no one was more qualified than Sukadeva Gosvami to give such advice to the great king. In reply, Sukadeva Gosvami told Maharaja Pariksit: "The highest perfection of human life, achieved either by complete knowledge of matter and spirit, by practice of mystic powers, or by perfect discharge of occupational duty, is to remember the personality of Godhead at the end of life. O King Pariksit, mainly the topmost transcendentalists, who are above the regulative principles and restrictions, take pleasure in describing the glories of the Lord. At the end of Dvaparayuga, I studied this great supplement of Vedic literature named *Srimad Bhagavatam*, which is equal to all the *Vedas*, from my father, Srila Dvaipayana Vyasadeva. O saintly King, I was certainly situated perfectly in transcendence [realized in the impersonal Brahman], yet I was still attracted by the delineation of the pastimes of the Lord [Krishna], who is described by enlightened verses. That very *Srimad Bagavatam* I shall recite before you because you are the most sincere devotee of Lord Krishna. One who gives full attention and respect to hearing *Srimad Bhagavatam* achieves unflinching faith in the Supreme Lord, the giver of salvation." (*Bhag.*2.1.610) "My dear Maharaja Pariksit, that great personality Srila Vyasadeva taught me this scripture, *Srimad Bhagavatam*, which is equal in stature to the four *Vedas*," (*Bhag.*12.4.42). Sukadeva Gosvami explained elsewhere that, "This *Srimad Bhagavatam* has elaborately described in various narrations the supreme soul of all that be the personality of Godhead, Hari [Krishna] from whose satisfaction Brahma is born and from whose anger Rudra takes birth." (*Bhag.*12.5.1).

Regarding the power of the contents of the *Srimad Bhagavatam regar*ding the creation of the universe, the secondary level of creation, planetary systems, protection by the Lord, the creative impetus, the change of Manus, the science of God, returning home back to

Godhead, liberation, and the summum bonum. (*Bhag*.2.10.1) After a full description of the contents of the *Bhagavatam*, Suta Gosvami explains that for the person who glorifies this *Bhagavata Purana* by chanting or hearing it, the demigods, sages, Siddhas, Pitas, Manus, and kings of the earth bestow all desirable things. By studying this *Bhagavatam*, a brahmana can enjoy the same rivers of honey, "ghee and milk" he enjoys by studying the hymns of the *Rig*, *Yajur* and *Sama Vedas*. A brahmana who diligently reads this essential compilation of all the *Puranas* will go to the supreme destination, which the Supreme Lord himself has herein described. However, not only can a brahmana who studies the *Srimad Bhagavatam* achieve firm intelligence in devotional service, but also a king [kshatriya] who studies it gains sovereignty over the earth, a vaishya who studies it acquires great treasure, and a shudra is freed from sinful reactions. Lord Hari, the supreme controller of all beings, annihilates the accumulated sins of the Kali age, yet other literature does not constantly glorify him. But that supreme personality of Godhead, appearing in his innumerable personal expansions, is abundantly and constantly described throughout the various narrations of this *Srimad Bhagavatam* (*Bhag*.12.12.6266). "From beginning to end, the *Srimad Bhagavatam* is full of narrations that encourage renunciation of material life, as well as nectarean accounts of Lord Hari's transcendental pastimes, which give ecstasy to the saintly devotees and demigods. This *Bhagavatam* is the essence of all *Vedanta* philosophy because its subject matter is the Absolute Truth, which, while not any different from the spirit soul, is the ultimate reality, one without a second.

The goal of this literature is exclusive devotional service unto that Supreme Truth" (*Bhag*.12.13.1112). "*Srimad Bhagavatam* is the spotless *Purana*. It is most dear to the Vaishnavas because it describes the pure and supreme knowledge of the *paramahamsas* [the swanlike saints]. This *Bhagavatam* reveals the means for becoming free from all material work, together with the processes of transcendental knowledge, renunciation and devotion. Anyone who seriously tries to understand *Sirimad Bhagavatam*, who properly hears and chants it with devotion, becomes completely liberated" (*Bhag*.12.13.18). Furthermore, the *Srimad Bhagavatam* has not always been a book but is an ancient work and has been a spoken tradition from time immemorial. This is illustrated by the following narration. Once Maitreya Muni began to describe to Vidura, saying, "Let me now begin speaking on the *Bhagavata Purana*," which was directly spoken to the great sages by the personality of Godhead for the benefit of those who are entangled in extreme miseries for the sake of very little pleasure. Sometime ago, being inquisitive to know, Sanatkumara, the chief of the boy saints, accompanied by other great sages, inquired exactly like you about the truths regarding Vasudeva, the Supreme Lord Krishna, from Lord Sankarshana, who is seated at the bottom of the universe. At that time, Lord Sankarshana was meditating upon his Supreme Lord, whom the learned esteem as Lord Vasudeva [Krishna]. For the sake of the advancement of the great learned sages who were there, he slightly opened his lotus like eyes and began to speak.

The sages came from the highest planets down to the lower region through the water of the Ganges, and therefore the hair on their heads was wet. They touched the lotus feet of the Lord, which are worshiped with various items by the daughters of the serpent king when they desire good husbands. The four Kumaras, headed by Sanatkumara, who all knew the transcendental pastimes of the

Lord, glorified the Lord in rhythmic accents with selected words full of affection and love. At that time Lord Sankarshana, with his thousands of raised hoods, began to radiate an effulgence from the glowing stones on his head. Lord Sankarshana thus spoke the purport of *Srimad Bhagavatam* to the great sage Sanatkumara, who had already taken the vow of renunciation. "Thereafter, Sanatkumara in turn, when inquired of by Sankhyayana Muni, explained *Srimad Bhagavatam* as he had heard it from Sankarshana. The great sage Sankhyayana was the chief among the transcendentalists, and when he was describing the glories of the Lord in terms of *Srimad Bhagavatam*, it so happened that my (Maitreya Muni's) spiritual master, Parashara, and Brihaspati both heard him. The great sage Parashara, as aforementioned, being so advised by the great sage Pulastya, spoke unto me this foremost of the *Puranas* [*Bhagavatam*]. I shall also describe this before you, my dear son, in terms of my hearing, because you are always my faithful follower (*Bhag.* 3.8.29). In this way, for thousands of years before the *Bhagavatam* was ever compiled by Srila Vyasadeva in a written form, it had been handed down and spread through an oral tradition. The *Matsya Purana* also says that which contains many narrations of spiritual instructions, begins with the *gayatri mantra (meditate, following up the OM mantra teachings, the technique is the same)*, and also contains the history of Vritrasura, is known as the *Srimad Bhagavatam*. Whoever makes a gift of this great work on a full moon day attains to the highest perfection of life and goes back to the spiritual world. All these references conclude that *Srimad Bhagavatam* is the most ripened fruit of the tree of Vedic knowledge consisting of the most clearly defined and highest realizations and understanding of ultimate reality the Absolute Truth. Over and above that it is also considered the incarnation of God in the form of sound vibration, as confirmed in the following verse: "This *Srimad Bhagavatam* is the literary incarnation of God, and it is compiled by Srila Vyasadeva, the incarnation of God. It is meant for the ultimate good of all people, and it is all successful, all blissful and all perfect," (*Bhag.* 1.3.40). From this verse it is made clear that *Srimad Bhagavatam* is meant for the benefit of everyone who is sincerely interested in the highest truth, regardless of their background. Furthermore, it is compiled by Srila Vyasadeva who was an incarnation of God. He appeared in this world in order to give people this knowledge for the highest good. After all, who can explain the characteristics of the Supreme better than the Supreme himself? This is also confirmed in *Bhagavad Gita* (15.5) in which Krishna explains that he is seated in everyone's heart and from him comes remembrance, knowledge, and forgetfulness. He is the knower and compiler of the *Vedas*, by which he is to be known. This is further elaborated in the *Vishnu Purana*, Book Three, Chapter 3: In every Dvapara [or third] age, Vishnu, in the person of Vyasa, in order to promote the good of mankind, divides the *Vedas*, which is properly but one, into many portions: observing the limited perseverance, energy and application of mortals, he makes the *Veda* fourfold to adopt it to their capacities; and the bodily form which he assumes, in order to effect that classification, is known by the name of Vedavyasa. Know, Maitreya, the Vyasa called Krishna Dvaipayana (Vedavyasa) to be the deity Narayana; for who else on this earth could have composed the *Mahabharata*. That form of Vasudeva composed of the *Rig, Sama,* and *Yajur Vedas*, is at the same time their essence, as he is the soul of *all embodied spirits*. He, distinguished as consisting of the *Vedas*, creates the *Vedas* and divides them by many subdivisions into branches. He is the author of those branches. He is those aggregated branches; for he, the eternal Lord, is the essence of true knowledge (*Vishnu Purana*, book 3, chapter 4). These verses clearly explain that it is none other than the incarnation of the Supreme Being who has appeared in this world to compile and divide the *Vedas* so that people of all levels of intelligence can understand them. It is explained that no ordinary person can do such a thing. How can people who are limited and finite understand the Unlimited and Infinite, unless that Supreme Being descends to explain this knowledge himself? Therefore, as stated in the above-mentioned verses, the essence of the Absolute Reality is found in the Vedic literature, especially within the *Srimad Bhagavatam*. Even though *Vyasadeva had worked for the welfare of all* by writing the many portions of Vedic literature, before he wrote *Srimad Bhagavatam,* he had still felt dissatisfied. This is a great lesson. Naturally, we all desire freedom from the problems that material life causes us, but only by engaging in direct spiritual activities does the spiritual living entity—the soul within these temporary material bodies—begin to feel any real relief or happiness (the experience is the key, soma).

How to do this by engaging in service or *bhakti yoga* to the Supreme Being is what the *Vedas* are ultimately meant to establish. Because this had not yet been prominently presented in the literature Vyasadeva had written, he was still feeling dissatisfied. Now he was trying to understand the cause of his dissatisfaction.

In all the literature compiled by Vyasadeva, there are many descriptions of the temporary universe, prayers to the demigods, the process for attaining one's material necessities, information about the soul, the Brahman, the supersoul, and the process of yoga for attaining spiritual realizations. There is also information about the

Supreme Lord, Bhagavan Krishna. But the detailed descriptions of God, his form, his incarnations, names, activities, potencies and energies, and how he is the source of everything, including the ever increasing spiritual bliss for which we are always looking, had not yet been fully described.

Therefore, although the spiritual truths are presented in different degrees, it could be asked why the Vedic literature seems to also recommend different processes for people to achieve various levels of material and spiritual perfection. This question was also asked by Uddhava in his conversation with Sri Krishna in *Srimad Bhagavatam* (11.14.1). He asked whether all the processes, recommended by the learned sages who know the Vedic literature, are equally important or if one process is superior. As is revealed shortly, there is one process that is more effective than others, but why there are different methods and rituals included in the Vedic literature is explained first. So in answer to Uddhava's question, as related in *Srimad Bhagavatam* (11.14.38), Sri Krishna replied that *the Vedic knowledge disappeared during the annihilation of the universe*. Then after the subsequent universal creation took place, He spoke the Vedic knowledge to Brahma. Brahma in turn taught this knowledge to his eldest son *Manu, along with the seven great sages* and Bhrigu Muni and other sons of Brahma who are associated with the creation of the universe. From these fathers of creation came many descendants who took the forms of demigods, demons, human beings, Guhyakas [spirits who have secret powers], Siddhas [a class of beings with all mystic abilities], Gandharvas [angel like beings], Vidyadharas [inhabitants of the heavenly planets], Caranas, Kindevas [demigod like humans on another planet], Kinnaras [similar to human beings but with a horse like body], Nagas [a race of extraordinary serpents], Kimpurusas [a race of extraordinary monkeys similar to humans], and so on. All of these species of beings had different desires and natures. To accommodate these different characteristics, there are many kinds of Vedic rituals, mantras and rewards. And due to the great variety of desires and goals among human beings, there are so many different theistic as well as atheistic viewpoints. Therefore, with their judgment clouded by the illusory energy, they all speak their own whimsical ideas of what is good for people without knowing the truth. From this we can understand that as various kinds of living entities evolved with different natures and desires, the Vedic literature also expanded to accommodate the different levels of consciousness. The *Vedas*, of course, are to provide the means by which the living beings can regulate their activities and thus be materially happy while simultaneously making spiritual progress. In this way, a variety of theistic philosophies have been handed down through tradition according to the level of illusion by which people are influenced. Everyone is essentially spiritual in nature, but as people forget their spiritual identity they become motivated by material desires for mental or sensual pleasure. Thus, people become engaged in a particular type of activity according to the mode of nature that influences them the most. Then they pursue a lifestyle or religious process that is conducive to the mentality they have developed. This is further explained in *Bhagavad Gita* (17.24): *depending on the nature into which the embodied soul evolves*, he develops a faith characterized by goodness, passion or ignorance. Men in the mode of goodness worship the demigods, those in passion worship demoniac beings, and those in darkness worship the departed and ghosts. *Bhagavad Gita* (9.25) also explains that those who worship demigods take birth among them, those who worship ghosts take birth as such, those who worship the ancestors go to them, *but those who worship Krishna return to him.* Herein we can understand that whatever mode of worship or activity we engage in brings particular results. Some may strive for happiness simply by filling their belly full of food and are content to work hard for no other reason. Others are satisfied by the pursuit for sex life, or by political power, or by religious activities, or by giving charity, or by achieving peace of mind. But if this is somehow or other based on pleasing the temporary body and mind of yourself or others, then all such happiness, being material, is temporary. The results are very meager, like trying to be satisfied with one drop of water while living in a desert. People who struggle to achieve one drop of happiness here and another drop there are busy running around, working very hard, and yet miss the real goal of life. This is explained in the *Bhagavatam* (11.21.28) by Sri Krishna that people dedicated to pleasures of the body that are obtained through the performance of Vedic rituals, or any other process for material happiness, cannot know him though he is situated in their hearts and the whole universe emanates from him. Such people are like persons whose eyes are covered by mist and cannot recognize what is right in front of them. In this way, according to the Vedic texts, people remain blind and cannot understand how to reach *the real happiness that exists within them* since they always focus on external comforts. Processes for attaining such things as external pleasures, heavenly bliss, a good future birth, or different levels of mystic awareness are included in the *Vedas* for those who want them. But such people miss the essence of the Vedic teachings that emphasize the need to reach the ultimate spiritual perfection. Ultimately, the Vedic system is to engage everyone in a process that will elevate them from whatever position they are in to a higher mode of living. Thus, there are many levels of understanding found within the Vedic tradition in order to accommodate the various forms of consciousness and tendencies of the innumerable living beings, especially humans. But without coming to the highest level of knowledge and realization, they will continue to engage in activities resulting in different degrees of anxiety and lamentation. Being concerned about this problem and foreseeing the troubled times ahead, the great sages five thousand years ago requested Suta Gosvami to explain the *Srimad Bhagavatam* after having learned it from Srila Vyasadeva and others. Thus they put forth the following request: O learned one, in this iron age of Kali men have but short lives. They are quarrelsome, lazy, misguided, unlucky, and, above all, always disturbed. There are many varieties of scriptures, and in all of them there are many prescribed duties, which can be learned only after many years of study in their various divisions. Therefore, O sage, please select the essence of all these scriptures and explain it for the good of all living beings, that by such instruction their hearts may be fully satisfied. (*Bhag.*1.1.–1011) In this way, the sages pointed out that in Kali Yuga, this present age, men are easily distracted by so many things and their lives are very short, so now let us not waste time but hear only the essence of all spiritual knowledge so that everyone can be satisfied and know the real goal of life and not remain confused. It was also for this reason that Srila Vyasadeva was feeling dissatisfied, even after compiling all the previous Vedic knowledge into written form in the earlier texts. The essence of all spiritual and metaphysical understanding and realizations had not yet been put into a concise and conclusive format. Vyasadeva, while questioning his unexpected dissatisfaction, was at that very moment greeted by the sage Narada Muni who had just arrived at Vyasadeva's cottage. Suta Gosvami, in *Srimad Bhagavatam*, Canto 1, chapters 5 and 6, relates the story in this way: Narada Muni asked Vyasadeva whether he was satisfied after having written the great *Mahabharata*. Sri Vyasadeva answered that in spite of all he had done, he was not content and, accepting Narada Muni as his spiritual master, questioned him about the root cause of the dissatisfaction he felt. Narada replied that the cause was that Vyasadeva had not written about the sublime characteristics of the Supreme. The philosophy that does not satisfy the transcendental senses of the Supreme is considered worthless, but that literature which is full of the transcendental descriptions of the name, form, and pastimes of the unlimited Supreme can bring about a revolution among the misdirected civilization of the world. Even though improperly composed, such literature is heard and accepted by saintly and intelligent men. This is exactly what is missing in the earlier Vedic texts as well as most other religious scriptures found in the world today. Narada is recommending that to include the topics he mentioned will certainly bring about a revolution to help all those who are living in a misguided civilization. The reason for this is simple: one may defend the science of religion or engage in so many philosophical conversations,

"But there will never be any final conclusion to such talks without practical experience of the Supreme. Without this genuine experience, all religious or philosophical talk is merely cultivated knowledge or mental speculation." Soma, soma, soma.

It is another way of passing time for the armchair philosophers because anyone, simply by juggling words or taking things out of context, can steer various controversial topics toward any conclusion they want. *This is the way some so-called religious leaders or propagandists use things like religion to justify their own selfish intentions.* More light is shed on these points in the *Bhagavatam* (11.22.56) wherein Krishna explains to Uddhava that when philosophers cannot agree on the way they view things; it is simply the interaction of Krishna's illusory energies that motivate their disagreements. But for those who have fixed their minds in Krishna, the Absolute Truth and ultimate conclusion of all spiritual realizations, the cause for argument and differences of opinion disappear. Just as when you may have several hungry people in a room discussing the various causes of and means to extinguish their pains of hunger, no one has to tell them that the process of eating a nice meal has worked when, after having done so, they automatically feel their hunger subside. *The experience is universal and, after eating and feeling satisfied, leaves no room for argument.* Similarly, after having reached the platform of experiencing the Absolute Truth, what need could there be for further argument or disagreement? The experience is universal for those who have reached it. And for those who have, participating in a religion or faith which condones the idea of deliberately quarreling or fighting wars with members of other faiths is utterly absurd. Indeed, such fighting only shows the gross ignorance of one's real spiritual identity and the animalistic qualities of such people, though they may claim strong allegiance to a particular religion. Of what use to the world is such a religion or philosophy? As pointed out in the *Manusamhita* (12.9596), such a religion is simply based on darkness and is worthless, producing no good reward after death. Therefore, to help avoid further quarrel and confusion among the people in this age, Narada Muni encouraged Vyasadeva to write and describe the eternal spiritual truths in a more direct manner. Narada explained to Vyasadeva that *spiritual knowledge, though free from material faults and connections, is still incomplete if devoid of an understanding of the transcendental characteristics of God.* But Vyasadeva, who is completely perfect, can meditate on the Lord's pastimes for the liberation of all people from material existence. Only one who has retired from activities for material happiness deserves to understand such spiritual knowledge and experience spiritual bliss. Therefore, *Narada emphasized that by Vyasa's mercy, those who are attached to material existence should be shown how to attain spiritual realization. Those who are truly intelligent will endeavor to reach this goal.* Vyasadeva knew all about spiritual knowledge and the transcendental qualities of the Supreme Being because he is a plenary portion of the Lord. Though he is birthless, he appeared in this world for the welfare of all. And to teach a lesson, he displayed dissatisfaction when he had still not engaged himself in writing the glories of the Supreme's spiritual qualities, and then accepted Narada as a spiritual master to learn the reason for his discontent. Thus, Narada continued to explain to Vyasadeva that learned men have concluded that the actual purpose for engaging in austerities, sacrifices, studying the *Vedas*, chanting the hymns, etc., is to advance in the knowledge of the transcendental characteristics of the Supreme, which is the only way to remove all difficulties. This is the ultimate process for perfecting one's life and for attaining full spiritual realization. This is the answer to Uddhava's question about whether a particular process in the Vedic literature is superior. Without understanding the Absolute Truth, one's knowledge of his real identity, or the universe, the purpose of life, and everything else in one's experience, is incomplete. So the conclusive purpose of the Vedic process is to increase one's knowledge of the Supreme, which will encompass all other forms of knowledge. The most direct way of doing that is through the practice of hearing about the Supreme Being from the Vedic literature, such as *Srimad Bhagavatam*. Simply hearing or studying this literature is a part of the process of bhakti yoga. As explained in *Bhagavad Gita* (11.54), only through bhakti yoga can one enter into the mysteries of understanding the supreme as he is. Similarly, *Srimad Bhagavatam* (1.2.20) points out that only by *bhagavata bhakti*, devotion to the Lord, can one get positive *scientific knowledge* of the Supreme Personality. Therefore, Narada requested Vyasadeva to describe the spiritual activities and qualities of the Supreme to satisfy inquisitive and learned men, and mitigate the sufferings of the people in general. After all, by engaging in ordinary yoga people may attain some peace of mind and freedom from desire and lust, but to give satisfaction to the soul requires the performance of devotional service, bhakti yoga, to the Supreme. This is the means of establishing a link between the soul and the Infinite Lord. This is what Vyasadeva had yet to do. And the perfection of this was to compile the great devotional work of *Srimad Bhagavatam*. Then when Sri Krishna had left this planet after performing his various pastimes by which he attracts the conditioned souls, and on the new moon night near the end of the month of Phalguna (February March), the planets aligned themselves in one direction above the Earth, with the planet Rahu over India. On that night in 3102 BC, according to the Vedic scholars, the world slipped into the depths of forgetfulness as Dvapara yuga ended and the age of Kali Yuga began. Shortly after this occurrence the great sage Vyasadeva had heard all these instructions from Narada Muni. The conclusion of this story, as related in the *Bhagavatam* (1.7.26), is that after Narada Muni had explained all these points, he took leave of Vyasadeva. Then Vyasadeva, in his cottage at Samyaprasa on the western bank of the

River Sarasvati, sat down to meditate. He fixed his mind, perfectly engaging it in devotional service, bhakti yoga, without any tinge of materialism, and thus he saw the absolute personality of Godhead along with his external energy, *maya*, which was under full control. *Deluded by maya, the living entities think they are a part of the material world and thus undergo the reactions of material miseries.* However, such miseries, which do not really touch the soul, can be counteracted by engaging in devotional service, bhakti yoga. But the mass of people do not know this, so to dispel their grief, materialistic infatuation, and fear, the learned Vyasadeva compiled this Vedic literature, *Srimad Bhagavatam*, which is in relation to the Supreme Truth. In this way, Srila Vyasadeva, the compiler of the original Vedic literature, wrote his concluding commentary on Vedanta in the form of *Srimad Bhagavatam*. In the *Bhagavatam*, Srila Vyasadeva very clearly establishes that real Vedanta, or the ultimate end of all knowledge, is to understand the supreme personality of Godhead, Lord Sri Krishna: In the revealed scriptures, the ultimate object of knowledge is Sri Krishna, the personality of Godhead. The purpose of performing sacrifice is to please him. Yoga is for realizing him. All fruitive activities are ultimately rewarded by him only. He is supreme knowledge, and all severe austerities are performed to know him. Religion [*dharma*] is rendering loving service unto him. He is the supreme goal of life. (*Bhag*.1.2.2829) Herein, it becomes clear that the aim of all austerity, penance, charity, scriptural study, *yoga practice, and religious activity is to regain one's love for God, Krishna*. Without that, all religious and pious acts, however positive and pious they may be, remain incomplete. Only through selfless love can God be captured or attracted, or can one bind oneself to him. From this study of all the Vedic literature and its purpose, it becomes clear that this is the real goal of all yoga and spiritual activities. This is what leads us to the heart of Hinduism, *sanatana dharma*, the awakened love for the Supreme Being and all other living beings, which are his parts and parcels. As the *Bhagavatam* explains, the practice of yoga or *karma yoga* alone is unable to cut the bondage of attraction to the illusory energy or worldly attachments. Therefore, the easiest way to achieve the most complete form of liberation is through the process of *bhakti*, loving attachment to the Supreme Being through devotional service, which can overtake all other forms of attachment. As we can see, the science of Vedanta is extensive and thorough. There is not much that it has not considered. It not only includes the knowledge of the Absolute Truth, but also explains the path by which one can attain his or her own individual realizations of the Absolute.

This in itself separates it from most religions we find today that usually do not include higher principles of spiritual self realization, but depend mostly on basic moral doctrines and the blind faith of the followers in their connection with the religious institution as the means of approaching God, or for being saved. The Vedic system, on the other hand, allows everyone individuality to take up the process in whichever way they feel is most appropriate.

The sages, gurus and Vedic texts provide the necessary insights and directions for progress, but an individual can work with full liberty of thought, and not on the basis of some institutional dogma. Thus, a person is allowed the freedom to explore the various avenues within the Vedic system to understand and perceive the Ultimate Reality and regain one's own relationship with God. *This divine knowledge is for the entire world, not merely some portion of it or for a certain class of people.*

These Vedic scriptures contain such a wide range of knowledge and information that can help one understand God and the process of realizing him that anyone from any background can find assistance by adding them to their life. These scriptures provide many descriptions of God, his beauty, characteristics, his pastimes and personality that are not available elsewhere. No matter whether one is merely inquisitive or is already a sincere devotee, these descriptions, especially from the *Srimad Bhagavatam*, can fill one's heart with the nectar of devotional love for the Supreme Being. Saints such as Shukadeva, who was already absorbed in the bliss of the Brahman, gave up that bliss to become absorbed in the devotional love of Lord Krishna in his pastimes in Vrindavana. And Shankaracharya, though he was the great preacher of *advaita* (nondualism) philosophy, appreciated the beauty and characteristics of Lord Krishna so much that he wrote the book, "Prabodha Sudhakar "in praise of Krishna. So these scriptures reveal the whole process from understanding the details of God's creation up to entering into the Divine bliss of devotional love for the most beautiful and loving Supreme Being. Within this process, as we can see, the worship of Lord Krishna and his expansions as Vishnu, Narayana, Rama, etc., is as old as the Vedic tradition itself. In fact, it is the essence of Vedanta according to the proposal and explanations of Srila Vyasadeva. So the conclusion of Vedic philosophy is essentially the doctrine of Vaishnavism, the worship of the personal form of God, especially as Vishnu or Krishna. The path of Vaishnavism is, basically, *sanatana dharma*, which is the practice of acting according to the eternal nature of the soul and reawakening our consciousness to our spiritual identity and the loving relationship we have with the Supreme. The Vaishnava *bhakti* movement has grown in many areas across India and beyond. It has also produced many volumes of devotional literature and poetry by numerous adherents in that tradition. The Vaishnava sect is one of the three major divisions of Hinduism, the others being Shaivism and Shakta. Vaishnavas have four major sects: the Ramanujas founded by Ramanujacharya; the Madhvas founded by Madhvacharya; the Vallabhas founded by Vallabhacharya; and the Gaudiya *sampradaya*, founded by *Sri Chaitanya Mahaprabhu who is regarded as an incarnation of Krishna himself.* Some of the aspects of following this Vaishnava philosophy are described later in this book. Essentially, a Vaishnava is a person who accepts Sri Krishna as the Supreme Being and worships him or any of his expansions or incarnations. The essence of Vaishnavism is expressed in the process of bhaktiyoga, unity with God through devotion. There is nothing more powerful than love and devotion to give one the impetus to absorb one's thoughts in thinking of another, the beloved. *Bhakti* puts less emphasis on ritual, austerity and sacrifice, and more on the *sadhana* and practice that can increase one's devotion. This is something that anyone can follow and develop, regardless of caste, status, background or disposition. *Bhakti* is not simply for Vaishnavas, but Shaivites also develop *bhakti* for Lord Shiva. However, Shiva does not reciprocate in quite the same way or in the number of ways of blissful exchange as does Lord Krishna. So the process of spiritual realization practiced by all Vaishnavas is bhakti yoga.

Elements of this devotional process are easily recognized in all other religions of the world, but bhakti yoga has been developed into a multifaceted science. Thus, all systems of philosophy and religion reach their culmination in Srila Vyasadeva's Vedanta, as specifically and conclusively described in the *Srimad Bhagavatam*. The main difference between the Vaishnava philosophy and all others of the world is that the goal is also the means of attaining the goal. In other words, *bhakti*, devotional service to the Supreme, is attained by engaging in devotional service to the Supreme. This devotional process of engaging in service to God refines and purifies one's consciousness to the level where he or she becomes completely spiritually realized, at which time a person knows his or her real spiritual identity. The Supreme also reveals himself to such a pure soul, and thus one's relationship with the Lord becomes awakened. Then *bhakti* is no longer merely a process to be followed, but it becomes a spontaneous flow of emotion and attraction for *the Supreme who reciprocates such love.*

Then the eternal, spiritual, loving activities and pastimes, along with a person's spiritual realizations and ecstasy, knows no limits.

If do you want to know more about the Vedas, seek information from: Abhay Charanaravinda Bhaktivedanta Swami Prabhupada, legacy, and those who spent their lifetime to commenting the holy vedas. My field of knowledge is in the teachings of use and correct approach to, Entheogenic substances in Tantric practices.

An entheogen, in the strict sense, is a psychoative substance used in a religious, spiritual or shamanic context. Tantra is an accumulation of practices and ideas, characterized by ritual that seeks to access the supramundane through the mundane, identifying the microcosm with the macrocosm. The Tantric practitioner seeks to use prana, and Vril power an energy that flows through the universe (including one's own body) to attain the so-called (soma) state, goals that may be spiritual, material or both. Most practitioners of Tantra consider mystical (Mystical experiences are in many ways the opposite of numinous experiences. In the mystical experience, all "otherness" disappear and the believer becomes one with the transcendent. The believer discovers that he or she is not distinct from the cosmos) experience imperative. Some versions of Tantra require the guidance of a guru. This book brings to you, the so-called practical guru's guidance. In this contest is sui generis. (is a Latin expression, literally meaning of its own kind genus or unique), I do hope this does clarify a little bit more about our field of work, the simple expression on divulgation of the vedas, also includes, an approach, to the holy practice of Bhakti yoga.

CHAPTER 7

Most Commonly Used Entheogens

OO-KOO-HE: *Following the main constituent of it, among others, like Anadenanthera peregrina (well know in the Colombian side of the Amazon rain forest, but, in the Brazilian side see Jababa)*

Family: Myristicaceae *Genus:* Virola, *Species:* Theiodora *Common names:* Cumala Tree, Parika, Yakohana Most, if not all, species of Virola have a copious red "resin" in the inner bark. The resin of a number of species is prepared as an hallucinogenic snuff or formed into small pellets. The most widely used species is thought to be Virola theiodora, a slender tree, twenty-five to seventy-five feet (7.5-23 m) in height, native to the forests of the western Amazon basin. The cylindrical trunk, 1 1/2 ft (46 cm) in diameter, has a characteristic smooth bark which is brown mottled with gray patches. The leaves (which have a tealike fragrance when dried) are oblong or broadly ovate, 3 1/2-13 in. (9-33 cm) long, 1 1/2-4 1/2 in. (4-11 cm) wide. The male inflorescences are many flowered, usually brown or gold, shorter than the leaves. The very small flowers, borne singly or in clusters of two to ten, are extremely pungent. The fruit is subglobose, 3/8-3/4 in. (1-2 cm) by 1/4-5/8 in. (1/2-1 1/2 cm); the seed is covered for half its length by a membranaceous, orange red aril. Members of this genus are mostly found in Amazonia and adjacent areas. Some species also occur in Central America. One species, Virola guatemalensis, can be found in southern Mexico and Guatemala.

At the beginning of time, Father Sun practiced incest with his daughter who acquired Viho by scratching her father's penis. Thus the Tukano received this sacred snuff from the sun's semen. And since its still hallowed, it is kept in containers called muhipunuri, or *"penis of the sun."* This entheogen enables the Tukano to consult the spirit world, especially Viho-mahse, the "snuff-person," who, from his dwelling in the Milky Way, tends all human affairs. Shamans may not contact other spiritual forces directly but only through the good graces of Viho-mahse. Consequently, the snuff represents one of the most important tools of the (Paje) or medicine man. Although about sixty different species of Virola are spread throughout the tropical forests of South America, and psychoactive principles have been found in at least a dozen species, it is only in the western Amazon and adjacent parts of the Orinoco basin that this genus has been used as the source of a sacred inebriant. The species most important as sources of the intoxicating snuff are V. calaphylla, V. calophylloidea, V. elongata, and V. theiodora, the last-named being without a doubt the most frequently employed. Yet locally, V. rufula, V. cuspidata, and other species may also supply the snuff. There are certain tribes—the primitive nomadic Maku of the Rio Piraparana of Colombia, for example—who ingest the red "bark-resin" directly, with no preparation, using B. elongata. Other tribes, especially the Bora and *Witoto*, swallow pellets made from the paste of the "resin," valuing for this purpose V. peruviana, V. surinamensis, V. theiodora, and possibly V. lorentensia. There is vague evidence that shamans in Venezuela may smoke the bark of V. sebifera "at dances when curing fevers "or that they may boil the bark and drink the liquor "to drive away evil spirits." Although the mythological significance and magico-religious use of Epana snuff indicates that it has been used since antiquity, the substance only recently began to receive attention from researchers. More creative natives, in some kind of secretive path, mixing, virola theiodora with fungi and tods secretions finally, gave birth to the fabled *oo-koo-he,* from the colombian amazon jungle they keep the formula secretive, like Jababa.

"Made famous by the hands of Terence McKenna who was born on November 16, 1946, and died on April 3, 2000, in Paonia, Colorado. At age sixteen, his family moved him to Los Altos, California to allow Terence to benefit from the highly rated California school systems. During his high school years, he was introduced to psychedelics. After graduating high school, Terence was enrolled at University of California (UC) Berkeley and was introduced to cannabis and subsequently to LSD. Experiences with psychedelic drugs would eventually be the base of his life's work. A knowledgeable human being who opened the eyes of millions of people around the world toward entheogenic substances, including myself, I do hope he is in an enlightened and much better realm, right now.

The earliest references to this entheogen dates back to the beginning of this century, when a German ethnologist reported on the Yelwana of the upper Orinoco area. It was not until 1938 and 1939, however, that the botanical association of Virola with the snuff was made. *The Brazilian botanist Ducke reported that the leaves of V. theiodora and V. cuspidata were the source of the snuff.* The first detailed description and specific identification of the snuff made from Virola was published in 1954 by ethnobotanist Richard Evans Schultes, in which its preparation and use among medicine men of Colombian Indians was described. Virola plant matter is used mainly by shamans among the Barasan, Makuna, Tukano, Kabuyare, Kuripako, Puinave, and other tribes in eastern Colombia. *The plant was employed ritualistically for the diagnosis and treatment of disease, and for prophecy, divination, and other magico religious purposes.* At one time, V. calophylla and V. calophylloidea were indicated as the species most valued, but later work in *Brazil* and elsewhere has established the primacy of V. theiodora as a source of snuff. Recent field studies have shown that the narcotic snuff is used among many Indian groups in Amazonian Colombia, the uppermost Orinoco basin of Colombia and Venezuela, the Rio Negro, and other areas of the western Amazon of Brazil. The snuff is apparently most highly prized and most deeply involved in aboriginal life among the various Indian tribes collectively called Waika in the upper Orinoco of Venezuela and the northern affluents of the Rio Negro of *Brazil*. These groups are variously named, but are most commonly known to anthropologists as the Kirishana, Shiriana, Karauetare, Karime, Parahure, Surara, Pakidai, and Yanomama. These tribes generally refer to the snuff as Epana, Ebena, Nyakwana, or some other variation of those terms. *In northwestern Brazil, this snuff and others are often generically known as Parica.* Unlike the Colombian Indians, among whom the use of the snuff is *usually restricted to shamans*, these tribes may use the substance in daily life. All male members of a tribe who are above the age of thirteen or fourteen may participate. The substance is often used in frighteningly excessive amounts and, in at least one annual ceremony, is consumed constantly over a two or three-day period. *Preparation:* Among the Columbian Indians, the bark is stripped from the trees in the early morning and the soft, inner layers are scraped. The shavings are kneaded in cold water for twenty minutes. The brownish liquid is then filtered and boiled down to a thick syrup which, when dried, is pulverized and *mixed with the ashes* of the bark of a wild cacao tree.

The various groups of Waika have several other methods of preparation. Those living in the Orinoco area frequently rasp the cambial layer of the bark and trunk and gently dry the shavings over a fire so that they may be stored for future use. When a supply of the sacred plant is needed, the shavings are wetted and boiled for half an hour or more, the resulting liquid being reduced to a syrup, which, after drying, is ground to a powder and finely sifted. This dust is then mixed with equal amounts of a powder prepared from the dried, aromatic leaves of a small plant, Justicia pectoralis var. stenophylla, which is cultivated just for this purpose. Then a third ingredient is added: the ashes of the bark of an Ama or Amasita (Elizabetha princeps), a beautiful and rare leguminous tree. The hard outer bark, cut into small pieces, is placed in glowing embers, then removed, and allowed to smolder to ashes. In more eastern areas of *Waika country in Brazil,* the preparation of the snuff takes place mainly in the forest. Trees are felled and long strips of bark are peeled from the trunk. A copious flow of liquid which rapidly turns blood red accumulates on the inner surface of the bark. After gently heating the strips, the shaman gathers the "resin" into an earthenware pot which is set on a fire. When the pot of red liquid is reduced to a thick syrup, it is sun dried, crystallizing into a beautiful amber red solid that is meticulously ground to an extremely fine dust like consistency. This powder *"Nyakwana snuff"* may be employed directly, but usually the pulverized leaves of Justicia are added "to make it smell better." The Bora, Muinane, and Witoto Indians of Amazonian Colombia and adjacent Peru use Virola not as a snuff, but through oral administration. They ingest small pellets or pills made from the resin to induce an intoxication during which the medicine men communicate with the "little people." The little people, I do call them green entities, they were the ones who a long time ago introduced me to the holy Vedas. These Indians utilize several species: V. theiodora, V. pavonis, and V. elongata, as well as possibly V. surinamensis and V. loretensis. The Bora of Peru also indicate that they have used a related myristicaceous genus, Iryanthera macrophylla, as the source of a narcotic paste for making the pellets. *The Witoto of Colombia* completely decorticate the trunk of a Virola tree. The shiny cambial layer on the inner surface of the bark which adheres to the bare trunk is rasped off with the back of a machete, and the raspings are carefully collected in a gourd. This material gradually darkens to a brownish red. The still-moist raspings are kneaded, squeezed repeatedly, and pressed over a wicker sieve. The liquid that oozes through, primarily composed of cambial sap, has a light "coffee and milk "hue. This liquid is quickly boiled without further preparation, possibly to inactivate enzymes which might destroy the active principles, and is then allowed to simmer, with frequent stirring, until the volume is reduced. When the liquid finally becomes pasty, the vessel is taken from the fire, and the paste is rolled into pellets for immediate use. *These pellets will keep their potency, according to the natives, for about two months.* When the pellets are not for immediate consumption, they are usually coated with a "salt," as the natives call it, which is a substance prepared from any variety of plants. The "salt" is always made through the same process. The plant material is first burned and *the ashes* are placed in a crude funnel made of leaves or bark. Water seeps slowly through the ashes, dripping out through a hole at the bottom to be collected beneath. The filtrate is then boiled down until a gray white residue or "salt" remains. The pellets of sticky resin are rolled in this powder. There is apparently a large assortment of plants employed for the manufacture of this "salt, "which the Witoto call Lesa. The lecythidaceous Gustavia poeppigiana is a common source of the ashes for filtration. The bark of the huge tree Eschweilera itayensis, of the same family, is also valued. An unidentified tree of this family, known to the natives as Chapena, is also sometimes used. The woody stump of a species of Carludovica or Sphaeradenia of the Cyclanthaceseae is reduced to ashes for this purpose as well. The leaves and fragrant inflorescence of the aroid Spathiphyllum cannaefolium give an ash which leaches out a high quality of "salt." The bark of a wild species of Theobroma, or several small palms, probably species of Genoma and Bactris, are similarly used. The Bora of Peru strip pieces of bark, only from the lower 4 to 8 feet of the trunk. The hard, brittle outer layer of bark is chipped off, leaving only the softer inner phloem. This later quickly turns brown from congealed oxidized "resin" and is vigorously pounded on a log with a mallet until it is shredded. These shredded sections are soaked in water with occasional kneading for half an hour or more, and then the pot is brought to a vigorous boil for another half hour. The bark material, squeezed dry, is then removed, and the remaining liquid is boiled and stirred constantly until only a thick paste remains. *Small pellets are then made from this paste for ingestion.* Fewer plants are used by the Bora for preparing the "salt" for coating the pellets: the leaves and stump of a species of Carludovica and a palm of the genus Scheelea being the primary of these. The psychoactive principles appear to be present mainly in the almost colorless exudate from the inner surface of the bark, which appears as soon as the bark is stripped from the tree. This resin like substance quickly turns reddish in a typical oxidase type reaction and then darkens, drying to a hard, glossy mass. In specimens dried for chemical study, this appears as a sticky, dark reddish brown gummy material. In many species this material contains tryptamines and other indolic compounds.

Observation of this process indicates that the reason for scraping the surface of the bark is to obtain all traces of the cambial layer that adheres to it. The medicine is prepared from the cambial sap, which is quickly boiled, causing coagulation of protein and possibly polysaccharides, and then simmered slowly to reduce the volume to near dryness. The whole process resembles that used for the isolation of natural products from the cambium of other trees; coniferin from gymnosperms, for example, except that ethyl alcohol or acetone are used rather than heat to destroy enzyme activity which might otherwise have an adverse affect on the desired products. *Medicinal uses:* The "resin "of Virola plays an important role in everyday native medicine: several species are valued as antifungal medicines. The resin is spread over infected areas of the skin to cure ringworm and similar dermatological problems of fungal origin which are so prevalent in the humid tropical rain forests. Only certain species are chosen for this therapeutic use, and the choice seems not to have any relationship to the psychoactive properties of the species. Indigenous peoples who are familiar with Virola trees from the point of view of their psychoactive potency exhibit uncanny knowledge of different "kinds "which, to a botanist, appear to be indistinguishable and of the same species. Before stripping the bark from a trunk, the tribesmen are able to predict how long the exudate will take to turn red, whether it will be mild or peppery to the tongue when tasted, how long it will retain its potency when made into snuff, and many other hidden characteristics. Whether these subtle differences

are due to the age of the tree, the season, the regional ecological situation, conditioning of flowering or fruiting, or other environmental or physiological factors it is at present impossible to say. However, there is no doubt concerning the tribesmen's expertise in recognizing these differences, for which he often has a very detailed terminology.
Effects: The effects of Virola snuff are said to be noticeable within minutes of initial use. One first experiences increased excitability, followed by numbing of the limbs, an uncontrollable twitching of the face, a lack of muscle control, nausea, and often vomiting. Macropsia-seeing objects in the visual field greatly enlarged—is characteristic of Virola snuff use, and this may contribute to the Waika beliefs about the hekulas, the spirits who dwell in the Virola trees and who meddle in the affairs of men. Shamans under the influence of the snuff often gesture and vocalize wildly, as they are in combat with these massive beings. The psychoactive effects of Virola snuff are thought to be a result of an *exceptionally high concentration of tryptamine alkaloids* present in the resin. Snuff prepared from Virola theiodora can have up to 8 percent tryptamine alkaloids. Two other alkaloids found in the resin act as *MAO inhibitors,* which allow the resin to have a psychoactive effect when consumed orally.

Schultes reported that the effects of the snuff were very intense and not at all pleasant. Shamans are reported to enter a dreamlike trance phase. *It has even been reported that a shaman died when under the influence of the snuff (snuffing is a bad idea, oral ingestion is much better)* possibly due to the very high amounts that are reported necessary to consume as snuff in order to achieve a state of trance. Sublingual consumption of the bark resin has resulting in relaxation and mild enhancement of the senses lasting several hours. This is possibly due to the potential for 5-MeO-DMT to be absorbed sublingually at low levels. The correct formula of the fabled oo-koo-he is kept secret to this day, above shows most of the plants used to prepare it. Jababa is the Brazilian version of the oo-koo-he. (this one I am pretty aware of the whole preparation process, which does imply, just lots of labor and having your hands in the right herbs, fruits, taxonomic kingdom, of frogs, etc.). Most the herbs are seasonal making difficult to partake with such sacrament.

Cannabis or (Cannabis sativa) Also known as *marijuana*, *marihuana*, and *ganja*, among many other names. Cannabis is indigenous to Central and South Asia and is known to have been used by the ancient Hindus and Nihang Sikhs of India and Nepal thousands of years ago. The major psychoactive chemical compounds in cannabis are *cannabidiol* and *tetrahydro cannabinol*. Cannabis, indica, ruderalis, sativa Americana. And about the lettuce that we eat in our salads. Neither of these two substances is truly vision provoking, but they have certain narcotic qualities which have been known and profited from for ages around the world.

As archaeology has verified, hemp was the first plant to be cultivated by human beings; in the Mediterranean was and is still used to extract vegetable fibers to make ropes and fabric, and for its entheogenous effects. Since ancient times, there have been recipes to eat it, to absorb its smoke, to drink it in teas, etc. As for the humble lettuce, it is fitting to mention that the white, milky latex that the plant secretes when it is ripe dries quickly and takes on an ochre color. It is this sharply bitter latex which makes the plant inedible when it is mature; it also contains the greatest number of narcotic ingredients known of and used in various mixtures cooked up by the pharmacists of yesteryear. All over the Mediterranean area, the use of lettuce by the people to induce a state of drowsiness in adults and children has been registered. In Spain, specifically, there is an old remedy of giving a pair of green lettuce leaves to children who cry at night so that they will fall asleep. Thus in the medieval centuries when witches were using complex psychoactive formulas, as in the current century, pharmacists used the same compounds with naturally similar effects. *The difference was that while the Holy Inquisition was burning witches, alive, pharmacists were backed up by the orthodoxy in power.* "The dark side stopping man, to reach awareness of God within "so, the next time you eat lettuce, remember "how useful such herb can be."

Salvia or (Salvia divinorum) among the most visionary plants ever experienced by man. Also known as *Diviner's Sage, María Pastora,* and *Seer's sage. Salvia divinorum* has a long and continuous tradition of religious use by Mazatec shamans, who use it to facilitate visionary states of consciousness during spiritual healing sessions. The known active psychotropic molecule of Salvia divinorum is known as *salvinorin A*. The psychedelic state salvia divinorum induces is quite similar to the "magic "mushroom experience only much milder and effects can last between sixty and ninety minutes. In higher doses, repetitive images with geometric or organic motifs may appear in the visual field. There are no known physical complications arising from the use of salvia divinorum and it is considered episodic rather than addictive. Salvia divinorum is reportedly used to positively benefit people choosing to explore their own consciousness. It can take you to the very edge and back amazingly quickly. This is what Salvia is known for producing—a very intense experience over a short time. It has been called the substance that *lets you see God on your lunch break!*

Ayahuasca (Banisteriopsis caapi) "see the chapter about ayahuasca." Ayahuasca, also known as *Caapi* or *Yage,* is a South

American jungle vine of the family Malpi–ghiaceae. It is usually mixed with the leaves of the *Psychotria viridis* plant and is used largely as a religious sacrament by indigenous tribes like the Urarina of Peruvian Amazonia. It contains *harmine, harmaline,* and *tetrahydroharmine.* These chemicals allow the primary psychoactive compound, *DMT* (from the Psychotria viridis plant), to be orally active.

Kanna or (Sceletium tortuosum) Kanna means, something to chew. The plant has been used by South African pastoralists and hunter gatherers as a mood altering substance from prehistoric times. The chemicals contained in sceletium tortuosum believed to possess psychoactivity include: *mesembrine, mesembrenone, mesembrenol* and *tortuosamine*. The species is considered as not threatened. It ranges from Namaqualand to Montagu through to Aberdeen and commonly occurs in quartz patches and is usually found growing under shrubs in partial shade. The plants are insect pollinated. Seed dispersal occurs during rain events by means of hygrochastic fruit capsules that open when wet, allowing seed to escape. The generic name *Sceletium* is derived from the Latin *sceletus*, referring to the prominent leaf veins that persist as the skeleton-like structure of the dry leaves. The genus contains eight species and is classified in the mostly weedy subfamily *Mesembryanthemoideae.* The genus is easily recognized by the persistent dry leaves that become skeletonized. In dry periods, these dry leaves enclose the young leaves, protecting them from harsh environmental conditions. The Afrikaans common name *kougoed* means something to chew. *Sceletium tortuosum* contains mesembrine and the related alkaloids mesembranol and mesembranone. Mesembrine is known for its effects on the central nervous system. The compounds also act as serotonin uptake inhibitors and in specified doses act as antidepressants, minor tranquilizers, and anxiolytics *used in the treatment of mild to moderate depression*, psychological and psychiatric disorders where anxiety is present, major depressive episodes, alcohol and drug dependence, bulimia nervosa, and obsessive compulsive disorders (U.S. Patent 6 288 104). Smith *et al.* (1996) review the data about *Sceletium* accumulated over three hundred years; they record the original folk methods for preparing Kougoed and document its psychoactive properties by reporting on the experiences of several test subjects.

Peyote cactus, or (*Lophophora williamsii*). *Peyote* is a small spineless cactus. It is native to southwestern Texas and through central Mexico. It is used worldwide as a supplement to various transcendence practices, including meditation, psychonautics, and psychedelic psychotherapy; and it also has a long history of ritualistic and medicinal use by indigenous Americans. Peyote contains a large spectrum of phenethylamine alkaloids, of which the principal one is *mescaline*. The name Lophophora comes from the Greek word for "crest bearer," referring to the tufts of hair that adorn the tubercles of some member of the genus. A number of species have been described, many based mostly on specimens in cultivation. They are now generally included in *Lophophora willamsii*. The legality of owning these cacti in the USA, or in other parts of the world, is questionable because of the local drug laws. This is unfortunate because it is an attractive cactus, and cultivated specimens don't contain enough alkaloid to make them a risk to the society.

Magic mushrooms or (Psilocybe) and Amanita Muscaria (muscimol). The *magic mushroom* is a genus of small mushrooms that grows worldwide. Hallucinogenic species of Psilocybe have a long history of use among the native peoples of Mesoamerica for religious communion, divination, and healing, from pre Columbian times up to the present day. *Psilocin and psilocybin are the hallucinogenic compounds* responsible for the psychoactive effects of many species in the genus. The ethno history of the Western Mediterranean basin shows the extensive use of the intoxicating mushroom *Amanita muscaria*. It's a well known, large mushroom, red on the outside with white spots. It has various popular names whose meaning itself is significant: the majority turn on the name wild bird in English it's known as fly agaric. Its psychoactive ingredient is *ibothenic acid* transformed in *muscimol* by the mushroom *drying process*. There are no traces of its consumption as part of a quest for sacred intoxication, but there is abundant evidence of its recreational consumption throughout history. Even today it plays an important role in the magic and child related iconography. This allows us to think of a prehistoric origin related to animistic practices and beliefs within a *shamanic cultural context* which has disappeared. For the majority of the present days, the intoxicating properties of this mushroom are unknown, and it is considered extremely poisonous. In spite of this, the tradition which relates *Amanita muscaria* to the hidden or magic dimensions of an unknown reality has persisted. Thus we see that the urban children of various countries even today continue to include mushroom iconography within the repertoire of children's drawings. It's normal in schools for children to draw red mushrooms in which they say that gnomes or elves live. By this I want to point out a noticeable cultural contradiction. On one hand, we're talking about a mushroom considered the most poisonous, but on the other hand people aren't disgusted by it they even greatly appreciate it. It's a warm and affectionate image which children often draw to represent the homes of the wonderful gnomes or elves of the forest. It's also common to manufacture things related to illusion, children's magic, or fantasy which have the basic shape and unmistakable color of *Amanita muscaria*. Those of us from that part of the world experience it as something deeply warm and familiar; gift and toy manufacturers know it and sell many objects with the image of this mushroom, even without knowing that it's an entheogenic mushroom. It's done by tradition. On these slides I'll show you some of the objects that anyone can find in a gift shop or a toy shop, In this sense, with *Amanita muscaria* a common phenomenon in anthropology is demonstrated. If they are sufficiently important, when sacred elements lose their central role for the society which kept them alive, they almost never just disappear into the depths of time and forgetfulness. Instead, the symbols and practices which made up the manifestation of sacred worship become a part of the recreational world of the society which had lived through it. This is a known phenomenon called "obliteration." Among the most significant manifestations linked to the traditional consumption of *Amanita muscaria* in the western Mediterranean is the Catalan expression "*estar tocat del bolet.* "This expression, "to be touched by the mushroom, "even today maintains an enormous vitality. In Catalonia, everyone knows what this traditional phrase means and it's applied to people whose behavior doesn't quite fit in with the accepted standards. But it's not a pejorative expression, like "to be drugged out" or "to be a nut." "To be touched by the mushroom "is a statement which implies friendliness and complicity in Catalonia it might be applied, say, to someone who's madly in love and who does cute little quirky things. Some years ago, I researched this subject and the results showed the relationship that exists between the psychological effects produced by the consumption of *Amanita muscaria* and all of the familiar cultural cosmos connected to it. In the course of this research I also found, much to my surprise, that the traditional consumption of *Amanita muscaria* in Catalonia and the south of France is not only reflected in symbolic and figurative carryovers, like those I just described. I also found some men who live in the Pyrenees Mountains, which separate France and Spain, who even today turn themselves over to the intoxicating effects of this mushroom sometime each year, when it appears in the fall in the birch and black pine forests. Of course they are neither old hippies nor people interested in entheogen, as I suppose are the majority of us here today. Instead they are European people who take them halfway on the sly because they know that "it might be forbidden," but who learned it from their grandparents and like to get intoxicated this way once in awhile. On the other hand, on the basis of various projects completed, we can affirm with little doubt that there is a direct relationship between *micophilic* societies and the territories where *Amanita muscaria* grows. With a few exceptions, in the European areas where this intoxicating mushroom doesn't grow, the traditional attitude of its inhabitants is one of *micophobia* and one of contempt and ignorance regarding mushrooms. It would take too long to discuss here all of the arguments which point to this parallel between the consumption of *Amanita muscaria* and *micophilia*. The fact that people who live in territories where *Amanita muscaria* grows know that if in the fall someone behaves irregularly after eating mushrooms it may simply be a case of accidental ingestion of *Amanita muscaria* or another intoxicating mushroom like *Amanita pantherina*, and that they don't worry in spite of rigid traditional taboos on its consumption, is significant enough. People who really appreciate mushrooms know perfectly well which ones are really poisonous and which ones aren't, whatever may be said. By the way, does make tea of it, is not safe, smoking with weed is the best way to experience with dry Amanita muscaria. (strong head experience mostly followed by the inner voice, who is a minor siddhis as mentioned before).

By the way, entheogens as seen above and below are common found all over the planet, not only in the amazon jungle, so *"the trees of knowledge are everywhere."* Most shrooms found in the Mediterranean are also found in the Americas, Asia, Africa and so on; Looks like those are the most common entheogen in the world sometimes, trading places with, common ones, like: "cannabis sativa." There are also others entheogenic mushrooms, Basically, I'm referring to *Psilocybe semilanceata*, a specimen whose active ingredient is *psilocybin*. We can conclude with reasonable certainty that *Psilocybe semilanceata* formed a part the psychoactive pharmacopoeia used in the popular culture of the medieval Spanish witches. (whom lots of them, were burned alive by, the Roman Catholic church), Indication of its probable use in this no longer existent context has been extracted from two objects used by witches in the fifteenth and the nineteenth centuries, medallions which bear the image of these mushrooms. They might also be linked to *pre-Christian practices of witchcraft,* from the fifteenth century and was found among various objects which the Catholic church of the epoch confiscated from women accused of witchcraft. As you can see, the devil appears in the form of an smiling face wearing long brown dresses and mostly burning innocent nice people alive, so the reason is, if you do experience with entheogen you no longer need such religion!. The *Psilocybe semilanceata*, belong to the family of entheogenic mushrooms well known and often consumed *in Central America* but, I do repeat, apart from these medallions there is no mention of its use either in Spanish documents about witches or in oral tradition. At most, the mushroom's popular name in Basque is also revealing: *sorguin zorrotz* ("witch's beak") which could refer to *the little nipple* which the upper part of the cap of this mushroom has, and to its consumption by ancient witches. Contrary to *Amanita muscaria*, *Psilocybe semilanceata* is widely known in the European Anglo Saxon world, where it has the significant popular name "freedom cap," an unmistakable reference to the mental effects which it produces. By the way I have no intentions to offend any neophyte from any crooked religion!

Blue Lotus or *(Nymphaea caerulea)*. Also known as the *Blue Egyptian water lily* or *sacred blue lily*. The original habitat of the blue lotus may have been along the Nile and other locations in East Africa, but it can also be found in the Indian subcontinent and Thailand. Nymphaea caerulea is purported to have a "divine "essence, bringing heightened awareness and tranquility. The known active psychotropic molecules for the blue lotus are the alkaloids *nuciferine and aporphine. In Egyptian mythology, Nefertem (possibly translated as the beautiful one who closes or the one who does not close; also read as Nefertum, Nefertem, Nefertemu) was originally a lotus flower at the creation of the world, who had arisen from the primal waters. Nefertem represented both the first sunlight and the delightful smell of the Egyptian blue lotus flower, having arisen from the primal waters within an Egyptian blue water lily, Nymphaea caerulea (This flower is widely used in Egyptian art, religion and literature. In much of the literature about ancient Egypt, it is called the "blue lotus." However, the true lotus, Nelumbo nucifera, was not found in Egypt until the time of the Persian invasion, when it was introduced as a food crop). Nefertem was an ancient sun god of Lower Egypt. He was important to various creation myths. Nefertem was associated with the young boy (Atum) who emerged from the lotus of Nun at the beginning of time. It was this boy that shed the tears from which all of mankind emerged. Due to this relationship, Nefertem was often called "the young Atum."* This particular entheogen only works mixed with other plants such as deadly night shade, etc., alone, I never felt any effect. Be extremely cautious dealing with belladonna, start with small doses of one hundred milligrams. Taking only one gram can be deadly to most people. Those two plants, when bundled, can be very visionary!

Iboga or (Tabernanthe iboga) Iboga is a perennial rain forest shrub and hallucinogen, and is the central pillar *of the Bwiti religion* practiced in West Central Africa, mainly Gabon, Cameroon and the Republic of the Congo, which utilizes the alkaloid containing roots of the plant in a number of ceremonies. Its main psychoactive constituent is the alkaloid, *Ibogaine*. Although the Iboga Tree Bark has been called the tree of knowledge in the past the vast body of research shows that the amazing plant can cure all addictions as well. Thus, it is really the *iboga tree of life.* One has to wonder why it is so vilified if it has such amazing properties. Conspiracies abound as to why this biblical herb is so hated by the squares in our society. Suggest that the government puts tens of thousands of people to work every day fighting the evils of the drug world. DEA, ATF, CIA, State DEA, attorneys, DAs, Judges, clerks, local police, etc. The estimate is 238,000 Federal and State jobs directly involved in the "fight" against drugs and 728,000 workers supporting them indirectly with office staff, equipment, weapons and vehicles, etc. Why not just cure the addictions and educate the masses to prevent drug abuse? (The dark side working against mankind, the evil power, which does influence the world.) Those same billions could be used to treat and educate, right? Do we really need to put everyone in jail? Suggest that once this powerful hallucinogen is taken the truth of life is seen on the Imax screen of your brain, forever altering the way you view the American treadmill. Mercedes, Acuras, Corvette, Rolex and the other trappings of success become just meaningless things. *(materialism sent man to the spiritual abyss, which mankind is facing now)*, Iboga Tree Bark renders the climb up the corporate ladder seem as useless as the climb up the mall escalator. This of course would result in the loss of billions of dollars worth of sales. You would finally love yourself the way God intended. Would American corporations benefit if you were completely satisfied with the skin you are in?. In the end is just greed of money, perpetrated from those 2 percent who not only influence but also control this world with their immense materialistic power, inflicting pain and suffering among billions of people.

> Three great forces rule the world: stupidity, fear and greed.
> —Albert Einstein

> The love of money is the root of all kinds of evil.
> —Jesus

> Nothing makes us more vulnerable than loneliness, except greed.
> —Thomas Harris

In the 1960s, a nineteen-year-old from the Bronx, Howard Lotsof, "accidentally" discovered that after dosing with ibogaine, his heroin addiction disappeared. Over a period of months spanning 1962-63, Lotsof administered ibogaine to nineteen individuals. Seven of them were opiate addicts attempting to get clean. All noted "an apparent effect on typical withdrawal symptomatology."

Syrian Rue or (*Peganum harmala*) also known as *harmal*. *Syrian rue* has been used as an entheogen in the Middle East, and in modern Western culture, it is often *used as an analogue of Banisteriopsis caapi to create an ad hoc ayahuasca*. The main active ingredient in peganum harmala is a fluorescent psychoactive indole alkaloid called *harmaline*. "Harmaga "or "*Syrian rue* "in Spanish. It's the famous Moroccan *hârmel*, from which comes the scientific name, *Peganum harmala*. The area where the most *P. harmala* grows and is consumed is in northern Africa, from Morocco to Syria in other words all along the southern part of the Mediterranean basin. Without a doubt, it was the most consumed entheogen in ancient times, as it is today. This plant also grows in Spain, and was used for various purposes which I will summarize. As you already know, the seeds of the *P. harmala* plant contain psychoactive *betacarbolinic* alkaloids in an enormous proportion which can reach 4 percent of its dry weight. Decades ago, it was discovered that one of these alkaloids, *harmine*, is exactly the same substance which *Banisteriopsis caapi, one of the elements of ayahuasca, contains*. This is a substance that I've been researching for years. Summarizing the various uses of *Peranum harmala*, one can say that *harmine chlorohydrate* is a narcotic used in current medicine to treat lethargic encephalitis. However, it also has other traditional therapeutic uses, as it has potent anthelmintic and sudorific effects; it is also used for physical and psychic tiredness. In Spain, until a few decades ago, they used to make a special wine from macerating Harmal seeds in normal grape wine. The goal of this process was to create a state of intoxication which was effective against depressed states of mind. Probably, this practice continues privately today. On the other hand, in Morocco and other places, there is a custom of boiling fifteen grams of the seed in a mixture of water and 30 percent lemon juice. After wards, this is dried in the sun and the resulting paste is smoked mixed with tobacco or cannabis, in order to reach a state of extreme sensitivity and *sexual energy*. Also in Morocco *P. Harmala* is used to make a famous shampoo which prevents baldness (and it seems that there really are very few bald Moroccans). It's also an important element in certain practices of witchcraft about which there has still been little research done. So *P. Harmala* plays an important role in the folk medicine of the areas where it grows, which indicates an old and probably semi sacred use in all of Northern Africa and part of Southern Europe (from Spain to Greece). This semisacred use, as I have commented, continues especially among the Moroccans and Arabs, where it is used by witches, and by people in general, to protect themselves from demon attacks. It is also used, significantly, to protect oneself from those who speak badly of others. Thus, from Morocco to Turkey the seeds of *P. harmala* constitute a sort of panacea sold by kilos in the market which also, apart from therapeutic uses, is especially used as a narcotic which provides states of intense happiness and a pleasant drowsiness. Currently, the most widespread way of ingesting the alkaloids of the *P. harmala* seeds but, especially by throwing a handful on the embers of the hearth fire and then throwing on top a piece of the mineral *Alumbre potásico* (*aluminum hydrate sulfate*), called *chépba* in Moroccan. Then the smoke produced by the combination is inhaled. Theoretically, the use of this mineral seems innocuous from a psychoactive point of view. It's a porous mineral and has a known bactericidal action. This explains why the Moroccans have the habit of putting a piece in the same container where they put the *P. harmala* seeds, perhaps to avoid bacterial contamination. However, there is no clear explanation as to its incineration. Maybe it's a good water-absorption diffuser and its use allows the seeds to burn more slowly; maybe because of its porosity it acts as an amalgamator.

Entheogen have played a direct role in the spiritual practices of countless cultures, but they are largely banned by governments and mainstream religions alike because they can alter your collective understanding of the nature of reality and your personal relationship with the divine, our father, who art in "Samadhi." Culture has consciousness all its own, and we both know that people function in this world as to what culture dictates. Our minds are bombarded by historical lies, violence, etc. Every time we turn on the TV, radio, read the news, etc., you will not be able to understand this kind of consciousness and its underlying purpose unless you break free from culture first; and this, among other things, is what an entheogen allows you to experience. It wipes off your cultural programming so that you can start with a clean slate and redefine your life according to your own rules, beliefs, principles, etc.

Following is a quotation from the Bible about that issue, if we can say that! By the way, another distortion from the Roman Catholic church or another lie? Probably both!

"But of the tree of the knowledge of good and evil, thou shalt not eat of it: for in the day that thou eatest thereof thou shalt surely die." It's not actually a physical death. The Bible is just referring to the death of the self "ego," which is usually what happens to you when you use entheogen. When you do dissolve your ego, enlightenment is achieved!

Much has been said and written about the use of entheogenic substances in the traditional American world. in *europeans* societies there has also traditionally been an abundant use of phytochemical resources to modify states of consciousness at will.

The problem with research in the Old World is that the majority of the traditions regarding the preparation of the entheogen and the identification of the specific substances used have been lost in the storms of modern history with the exception of alcoholic drinks. There, we don't have at our disposal exotic ethnic minorities like in North and especially *in South and Central America, with their shamans,* the old wise man who knows about medicinal plants, and the woman of the tribe who knows the secrets of their preparation. Europe, is recovering knowledge about the entheogenic substances used in ancient times, but all traces of the popular rites in which entheogenic substances were consumed have been lost. We only know something about the most famous ancient rites, like the Greek ones of *Eleusis (see the road to Eleusis from Wasson/Hofmann/Ruck, nice book)* and Samoth race. In other words, in Europe the traditional use of entheogenic substances has only survived in very, very marginal places where there are still some elderly people of the mountainous regions who take them in a recreational, individual way. Of course, I'm not referring here to the new generations interested in the subject, the majority of whom are a product of the psychedelic experience of fifty years ago, and not of ancestral traditions, the 1960s. For this reason, I would make a quick presentation of such substances with psychoactive potential most habitually used in the ancient traditions of the European world I'm not going to talk about the consumption of alcoholic substances or tobacco. There's already a lot written about that. So let does show couple more entheogens as follow below.

"Devil's tomato" or "Moorish weed," *Solanum villosum*. This plant is often mistaken for *Solanum nigrum*, and often comments are made about the two without the pertinent, and very necessary, distinctions. *S. nigrum* bears some relatively appetizing and sweet black fruits, although it sometimes takes on an orangish or brown color which causes the historical confusion between the two varieties. The gluco alkaloid contained by different types of Solanum found in the wild gives it its sweetish flavor as well as a slightly narcotic effect which has made adolescents of various epochs consume it with delight. One of the varieties of Solanum is *S. lycopersicum*, known universally for its bright, red fruit: the tomato. About *S. villosum*, we can only say that it contains psychoactive ingredients much stronger than its cousins, and that its effects were known by the classical Greeks and Romans. The Roman writer of the first century, Pliny the Elder, left us a work about plants in which he states that he doesn't want to say anything about *S. villosum* because he "deals with remedies and not with poisons "but he adds mischievously for the knowledgeable and the curious that a *few drops of the juice of this plant are enough to disturb one's reason.* He also notes that the ancient Greeks used this plant as an entheogen: "It's said," affirms Pliny, "that a dose of one drachma (a unit of apothecary weight equal to an eighth of an ounce or to sixty grains), provokes lascivious imaginations, fantastic visions which seem real; a double dose, a real craziness; and whatever greater dose, *death*." [1/8 of an ounce = 3.5 grams], never ever start with three grams start with one hundred milligrams and rise up the dose in steps with caution, until reach the right amount of it, what is good for you, is not to somebody else.

Recently, I've been able to gather some testimony about a final carryover of the consumption of this entheogen on the famous island of Majorca, and I don't know whether it could also be found in the other Balearic islands. Some Majorcan peasants keep the berries of *S. villosum* in closed jars and they recommend insistently not to consume "Devil's tomato" even though they store it. This attitude shows their tacit knowledge of and their interest in the use of these fruits since, naturally, if it weren't the case they wouldn't go to the trouble of drying and storing the berries.

"*Datura family, particularly Datura estramonium.*" This plant family is sister to the American Brugmansia, with which you are already familiar. In Spanish, *Datura estramonium* receives the significant popular names of "hell's fig," "devil's eggplant," and infinite others which include many references to craziness, devils, and saints. "*Datura estramonium*" was very widely used in the sacramental traditions. It's a big plant which reaches a height of one and a half meters. It grows in the little cared for gardens of all of the Mediterranean basin, near the waste dumps, and even on the most heavily frequented beaches next to the more fashionable bikinis and suntan lotions. It characteristically has white, bell shaped flowers, green prickly fruits, and an especially strong medicine smell. It can be said that *D. stramonium* is one of the few existing hallucinogenic plants, in the strict sense of the word, since its consumption produces a modification of consciousness so strong that it leads to a total loss of contact with the environment. It contains *l*hyoscyamine, reaching up to .5 percent of its dry weight; this alkaloid tends to be found transformed into atropine. Beside this, both alkaloids are commonly found accompanied by a certain amount of scopolamine. Due to the high proportion of alkaloids which it produces, stramonium has been often used in medicine, especially as a hypnotic and in the treatment of asthma. Until this century, cigarettes made from the leaves of stramonium were the most effective known remedy for a persistent cough or asthma. If we speak about the history of stramonium, it can be said that it has a confusing origin. On one hand, it was one of the most frequently used psychoactive ingredients used in the brews cooked up by European witches; according to some authors, it originally comes from the lands near the Caspian Sea, in the Near East. On the other hand, some researchers claim that it's a plant of Mexican origin, which didn't enter Europe until 1577, through Spain. If the second hypothesis is true, we would have to conclude that the consumption of stramonium spread with a strange and extraordinary rapidity through European folk and magical culture. I won't insist any more on detailing this argument about its origin, but it is important if it really is a Mexican plant brought to Europe during the first voyages of the colonial epoch, it would imply that in Europe there was a network of exchange of knowledge about entheogen much more solid than is supposed today. The physical effects of atropine and hyoscyamine are very intense and now I'll describe them in detail. You all probably know that both alkaloids begin by paralyzing the vagus, the trachea, and the nerves of the involuntary nervous system. The visions and psychoactive effects associated with stramonium are probably related to this paralysis of the parasympathetic nervous system. Without a doubt, it's due to its high toxicity that *Datura estramonium* is generally ingested by people through their skin and through their mucous membranes. In some cases, the plant's raw sap is used; in others, ointments are elaborated with this and other plants. It was this second system application which generated the old image of the witch flying on a broomstick: effectively the European women rubbed the stramonium based potions that they brewed into their *vaginal mucous membranes, using a stick for intravaginal application.* Since the intoxication appears within a few moments, the women felt the sensation that they were flying while riding the stick. On the other hand, the visions induced by the consumption of stramonium are more related to experiences of flying than other psychotropic substances. It produces an intense sensation that the intoxicated individual is flying in other dimensions of reality where he or she encounters new people and situations, but one especially gets the feeling of being able to know what is happening in faraway worlds. That's why the Inquisition Tribuna, often accused European witches of knowing of events that had happened far away from them, and that this could only be done with the help of the Devil which was a good reason to burn them alive. (Another atrocities done by the Roman Catholic church) Meanwhile, the witches claimed to have this knowledge thanks to the secrets of the potions that they used. With reference to stramonium, there's another important aspect to comment on. The complex psychoactive compounds used in Europe between the thirteenth and nineteenth centuries demonstrate an important accumulation of knowledge referring to the use of entheogens; besides the psychotropic substances, they used activating elements like soot and coal, and regulatory and purifying substances like wild celery, parsley, and cinquefoil to counter the toxicity of certain natural entheogens. *Is said in Hindu tradition Lord Shiva used Datura, cannabis, shrooms, among others entheogens, if God uses why not us? Some fools think they are more knowledgeable then God, when they do outlaw such substances!*

"Belladonna, Atropa Belladonna." It also was much used as an entheogen in Spanish witchcraft traditions and in Europe in general. In Spain its use was very well known, in spite of the rarity of this solanaceous plant in the Iberian Peninsula, where it only grows in the beech and oak forests of the Pyrenees and pre Pyrenees areas. Its leaves contain a great quantity of potent psychoactive substances (like *hyoscyamine and atropine*), and have historically been another of the substances most *used to modify states of consciousness* from the central Europe. Thus, for example, the wise man Dioscorides of antiquity affirmed that drinking the extract of the quantity of belladonna that fit in a *drachma (the Greek coin)* caused one to enter into states of insanity and to experience certain pleasant imaginations which could be understood as if they were dreams. Inebriety by belladonna was also frequent among adolescents in the European places where it grows, as they used to eat its sweet fruits which are similar to grapes. Another detail which gives an idea of its importance is that in Spain (in spite of its relative scarcity), it was so widely used in traditional pharmacology that there is even a current Ministerial Order, from the year 1949, which prohibits the gathering of wild belladonna. And I'm talking about sixty years ago, when there still weren't any prohibitions on the consumption of entheogens. I've already commented on the way that atropine and hyoscyamine act: it paralyzes the involuntary nervous system, but apart from this, belladonna also dilates the pupils a great deal, and the eyes acquire a brilliant and very pretty tone. This is where the popular term "belladonna" (which means "beautiful girl" in English) comes from, as this plant was christened in Italy in the Middle Ages. There it was used as a *feminine cosmetic to enhance one's eyes*. In Europe there are plenty of old and very funny stories which talk about the use of this entheogen by women to satisfy themselves sexually, cheating on their husbands with men who appeared to them in visions after having taken belladonna. With reference to belladonna alone, writings have been found which speak of *grinding between 30 and 200 milligrams of dry leaves, or between 30 and 120 milligrams of the root, and then later ingesting it orally or smoking it (smoking has small effect)*. Nevertheless, the majority of the information conserved about the use of belladonna *speaks of it as one of the active components used in combination with others to create complex entheogenic potions*. As I've mentioned before, in these mixtures, entheogenic substances were included with other detoxifying and regulatory substances. As you see, can contains six different entheogens, as well as other plants which are probably stabilizers and potentiators of the effect. The powerful visionary deadly nightshade is one of the most visionary plants of light who I ever had the opportunity to experience with. I've had seen many followers of Michel de Nostredame talking on TV about Nostradamus predictions. If they have the balls to use that plant they could foresee the future like him, I've no doubt about that! But there is a catch, if they do not prepare themselves right and have the knowledge to use the right amount, they will end up meeting him in the afterlife! That is a powerful plant who we cannot mess around with, one mistake we make, "the cemetery we go." Some folks on other books do recommend two grams, that dose to some people is enough to kill so, be cautious, I do recommend start with one hundred milligrams and step by step reach maximum of one gram even though the decision is yours, ayahuasca is strong, like, mushrooms, Jababa, oo-koo-he, etc., but that plant has poison in it!, why is so dangerous. But if you have the balls to use it like I did you can see the future like me. My experience last for one whole week I got very close to die.(the visions who I saw are not pleasant does foresees a catastrophic destruction of many cities, around the earth, triggered by natural sources "polar shifts" culminating in failure of the economic systems leaving our planet vulnerable to another great war with immense devastation of life, unfortunately the beautiful big city of New York, will be under the water, "Arc de Triomphe" and the surrounded of many cities as like, level down, so this is the reason, why I urge with immense focus, to people seek better level of consciousness, before is to late!, the meaning of this book is not predict the future so, I will no longer embrace this topic, see the future is not the scope of my work) remember if one man can do another can too, what do you need is the correct knowledge to avoid trouble, don't be afraid, by the divine grace and love of God our souls never ever die, I saw death face to face, so be careful go with well-established entheogens without poison, let us play safe, life can be nice so, let's leave longer lives. The meaning of this book is to teach you how to use "plants of light "and being alive not dead. I do have more than twenty-five years of practical use not theoretical but, practical, that is what makes the difference, in the beginning I made mistakes but I was lock, my knowledge in this field is my gift to you, if you are patience you can make it without troubles. Never sub estimate the wise man! In the path to gain knowledge. Inexperienced neophytes can end up dead, most did it, so let learn from those who made it and still alive. I go further, I read one book, where one so-called psychonaut does recommend the use of three hundred seeds of morning glory, or Hawaiian baby wood rose; if you do so, you can end up dead or in the madhouse. I do recommend maximum to the first timers four seeds, not three hundred. So they really did what they say they do? How can they recommend such dose? Let's be positive, well-established entheogens are safer than such seldom-used herbs. The tincture of belladonna leaves used to be one of the most popular poisons among professionals. It was believed that the famous Roman poisoner Locusta killed the Roman emperor Claudius with her deadly weapon a tincture of belladonna. Salvia is visionary, mostly opens the third eye, belladonna mixed with blue lotus and cannabis does show you the future, again Goithyja must say, cautious is advised.

Opium, Papaver somniferum. The plant is commonly known in Spanish as "dormidera," which comes from the word for sleep (unlike the English word "poppy"), and it is thus differentiated from the resin, which is known as opium. I don't want to go into too much about this specimen because it's already universally known. I only want to remind you that *Papaver somniferum* is the natural source of the multiple opiate derivatives which we know, and that its applications are so extensive that it practically deserves the title of "sole medicine." The resin of the poppy contains an extraordinary quantity of alkaloids not only in variety, but in amount. According to Wehmer, the *narcotine* and morphine together account for 16 percent of the weight of *Papaver*, and all the other alkaloids add up to another 1 percent. From a historical point of view, the use of poppy goes back to the year 3000 BC, when it seems that it arrived in Greece from a more Eastern location. The white flowered variety of the poppy, which produces smaller capsules than the red variety, And until the second half of the twentieth century, it was very common to plant various poppy plants in family gardens for the family's own use. It was taken to fight insomnia, toothache, and earaches; it was also used to calm children when they cried too long, and as a general analgesic. In some European countries even today it is common to use the seeds to decorate homemade cakes, also, until recently, poppy was taken for intoxicating and narcotic purposes. Presently there are many peasants who continue cultivating poppy for their own consumption, but they know that it's forbidden and they hide it. If the Spanish police discover a garden with some opium plants, they don't usually do anything to the farmer; they only tell them to pull them up because there are addicts who could come to steal them and that's it. On the other hand, if the same police find a young person with this little plantation, they might even turn him or her over to a judge. In spite of all this, the primary use of opium as an intoxicant occurred, and still occurs today, in Turkey (despite current strict prohibition), Iran, and ex-Yugoslavia and of course its consumption increases even more if we turn to the countries of the Middle and Far East. It Does make me recall also the sacrament taken a long time ago in Geece "The Eleusis Mysteries" kind of powerful wine content, mixed with herbs, like cannabis, opium, blue lotus etc, the exact mixture to this day is a mystery, if rebirth is given to such substance in Greece the same prosecution may happen.

Henbane, or "crazy weed," *Hyoscyamus niger L.* Like other entheogens which have the same vision provoking potential, henbane contains l-hyoscyamine converted to a greater or lesser degree into atropine and scopolamine. It's another of those plants which have been used as an intoxicant throughout the history of the Old World. This is due to its wide spontaneous geographic diffusion, since it's very easy to cultivate. Its wide diffusion was also probably favored by the fact that the alkaloids penetrate directly through the skin and the mucous membranes, facilitating its administration. As for its physiological and psychoactive effects, I won't repeat them, but they are the same ones that I've already described when speaking *of belladonna and stramonium. Henbane also produces a special sensation of great corporeal lightness, of losing weight to* such a point as to be able to float in the air at will. This sensation is so vivid that it was also immortalized by the same legends of flying witches. Henbane was probably the plant most used as an entheogen in medieval European witchcraft traditions. There are lots of funny stories about its use by the people as an intoxicant and as a soporific there's a saying in Spanish that "he who eats henbane won't go without sleeping." To recount just one anecdote about it, I'll explain that during the long medieval centuries, the Gypsies used to throw henbane seeds on the coals in the public bath houses to get the bathers into a stupor and steal their purses. Like the other entheogens that I have mentioned, henbane has often been used as a remedy for the treatment of diverse pathologies because it mitigates physical pain, causes forgetfulness, and calms spiritual pain by submerging the intoxicated subject in complete unconsciousness. For this very reason there are words in Spanish derived from the Spanish word for this plant, such as "embeleñar" and "embelesar," which mean to suspend, seize, or captivate someone's senses for whatever reason. There are also some linguists who maintain that the Spanish word for poison, "veneno," comes from this plant. The common word for *Hyoscyamus* seems to be rooted in the name "Belenos," a Gallic divinity who liked to take henbane very much. In Egypt henbane also appears in the Eber Papyrus, in the year 1500 BC, and it is suggested in various works that the *priestesses of Delphos made their prophecies while intoxicated by henbane smoke probably also ethylene gas.* The Greek author Plutarch, in the first century CE, wrote about the Oracle (also known as the Pythia), a succession of priestesses of Apollo who figured prominently in Greek culture for over a thousand years. Plutarch described how a woman would enter a small chamber (adyton) in the temple of Apollo and inhale sweet-smelling vapors (pneuma) from a fissure in the mountain before entering a trance. From this state, she would provide responses to seekers'

The toad, *Bufo* sp. The use of this animal for entheogenic ends has also been reported in South America. Its glands contain a substance called bufotenin which is still used today in medicine as a hallucinogen. Throughout the middle ages, this was another natural chemical resource which was known and used by witches. Some detailed references to the use of bufotenin appear in the accusations of five witches of Fago (in Aragon, Spain) tried around 1657. From some notes written about the trial held by the Inquisition before deciding whether to burn them alive or not, the following was extracted: "the accused said that she had a toad and they whipped it with heather branches, they took what they made it squirt out, they rubbed themselves with it and went wherever they wanted." In Catalonia, a present-day carryover of the human use of toads remains. Until only forty years ago in the Pyrenees range a form of popular justice called "sandbagging" was applied. This consisted of punishing petty delinquents in the very villages where they were caught, without the necessity of turning them over to regular justice. To carry out the punishment, a woman's stocking was filled with sand, and the convict was beaten with it on the back and chest for a preset time. This way, the convict was left sore for several days without causing serious wounds. But if the punishment deserved was greater, the villagers put a live toad in the stocking with the sand; this left the convict not only with the physical pain of the blows, but also made him or her forget what had happened during those hours and gave possibly terrifying visions which augmented the punishment. (Stressful situations can unchain bad experiences.) Curiously, among the parts of the body where the thick liquid extracted from the toad was applied, the genitals never appear. It's strange because this part of the body is the point of greatest physiological absorption and is where witches applied the rest of the ointments which I've mentioned. I've never tried it, but probably bufotenin is fairly irritating and it may even go so far as to cause pain, which would be why it was never applied this way in spite of its toxicity. So I could mention many more entheogens, but the true meaning of this book is prepare the neophyte to experience with entheogenic substances not lay hundreds of plants, fungi, toads, etc, down. if you still seek more info about all those entheogens you can find on many books written in that subject. Before I finish this chapter let's talk about baby wood rose, and little more about entheogenic substances also from frogs.

Giant leaf frog (Phyllomedusa bicolor) is a hylid frog found throughout the *Amazon jungle* of northern Bolivia western and northern *Brazil*, south eastern Colombia, eastern Peru, southern and eastern Venezuela, and the Guianas. Locally, this species is now jeopardized by biopiracy because it produces a waxy secretion that may have medicinal uses against AIDS, cancer, and other diseases. The Matses and Mayoruna people apply the poison of the frog to self-inflicted burns in order to enter an altered state of consciousness. The poison has been reported to produce a variety of effects ranging from stimulation, to sedation, anorexia, and hallucinations. The poison contains dermorphin and deltorphin which act on opioid receptors. Also the Phyllomedusa bicolor, otherwise known as the Sapo, in Portuguese language. Traditionally, the Mayoruna tribe uses this frog's gooey secretions to gain superpowers, First they tie the frog up and scare it into releasing its venom. Next the natives burn little holes in their arms or self-inflicted burns, and rub the venom into the wounds. Then they get nauseated and sometimes vomit for half an hour, and then they experience also a sharpening and heightening of the senses and an ability to go for days without food or water. There are also species of frogs yet to be classified only know by the natives of the Amazon rain forest.

I've seen a yet unclassified species of tiny little frogs highly poisonous, before. If you hold such frog with your bare hands they do release a "venenum "who gets into the blood stream throughout the skin finding shelter in the liver of the recipient, if not treated in couple days the "venenum "keep on dissolving the liver until death, occurs, one scientist from Brazil many years ago died dealing with such frog.

Hawaiian Baby Woodrose (Argyreia nervosa) is a perennial climbing vine, also known as Elephant Creeper and Woolly Morning Glory. This plant is a rare example of a plant whose hallucinogenic properties have only recently been discovered by non-Hawaiians. While its cousins in the Convolvulaceae family, such as the rivea corymbosa ololiuhqui and ipomoea violacea morning glory, were used in shamanic rituals of Latin America for centuries, the Hawaiian Baby Woodrose was not traditionally recognized as a hallucinogen. Its properties were first brought to attention in the 1960s, despite the fact that the chemical composition of its seeds is nearly identical to those of the two species mentioned above, and the seeds contain the highest concentration of psychoactive compounds in the entire family. Hawaiian Baby Woodrose seeds contain LSA (dlysergic acid amide), a precursor to LSD. The seeds are generally eaten, although there are a variety of preparation methods used. The active oral dosage ranges from four to twelve seeds and lasts from six to twelve hours. The LSA content of Argyreia nervosa is 0.14 percent of the dry weight of the seeds. Side Effects and Adverse Reactions: Some users commonly report experiencing anxiety, nausea, gas, vomiting, and abdominal cramps. Delirium, dizziness, confusion, paranoia, fear, and panic are less common, but sometimes experienced with higher doses. I do consider taking twelve seeds a high dose, the ideal is, take four seeds.

Lets try to better understanding of the terminology, Entheogens, Psychedelics. The general group of pharmacological agents commonly known as hallucinogens can be divided into three broad categories: psychedelics, dissociative, and deliriant. These classes of psychoactive drugs have in common that they can cause subjective changes in perception, thought, emotion and consciousness. Unlike other psychoactive drugs, such as stimulants and opioids, the hallucinogens do not merely amplify familiar states of mind, but rather induce experiences that are qualitatively different from those of ordinary consciousness. These experiences are often compared to nonordinary forms of consciousness such as trance, meditation, conversion experiences, and dreams. One thing that most of these drugs do not do, despite the ingrained usage of the term hallucinogen, is to cause hallucination. Hallucinations, strictly speaking, are perceptions that have no basis in reality, but that appeared entirely realistic. A typical "hallucination" induced by a psychedelic drug is more accurately described as a modification of regular perception, and the subject is usually quite aware of the illusory and personal nature of their perceptions. Deliriants, such as diphenhydramine and atropine, may cause hallucinations in the proper sense. Psychedelics, dissociatives, and deliriants have a long history of use within medicinal and religious traditions around the world. They are used in shamanic forms of ritual healing and divination, in initiation rites, and in the religious rituals of syncretistic movements such as União do Vegetal, Santo Daime, and the Native American Church. When used in religious practice, psychedelic drugs, as well as other substances like tobacco, are referred to as entheogens. An entheogen, in the strictest sense, is a psychoactive substance used in a religious or shamanic context. Entheogens generally come from plant sources which contain molecules closely related to endogenous neurochemicals. They occur in a wide variety of psychedelics of various religious rites and have been shown to directly provoke what users perceive as spiritual/mystical experiences. After talking about shamanism & tantra I would mention also, the preparation, in steps to follow up, before, during and after the spiritual/mystical experience it self.

CHAPTER 8

Tantra and Shamanism

Shamanism and Tantra, how are they alike? How are they different? Why and how do they fit together? The shamanic path and the Tantric path are both very old and based on indigenous cultures that were nature and goddess based. Ancient peoples who lived in both these ways were close to the earth. They believed that the earth was the Great Mother to whom they owed their very existence and to whom they could count on.

Similarities

Both paths rely heavily on the idea that everything is energy and that one can learn to see, feel, touch, and know the energetic world. Both paths embrace freedom, say yes to all you are, with consciousness. Walk impeccably and love yourself as a divine being. Both paths understand the fundamental nature of the balance between the male and the female with no one gender better or worse than the other. In both paths, the overall concept of ayni—to live in harmony with a balance of give and take—prevails. Both paths believe that everything is divine. *There is no evil except in the hearts and minds of humans.* Both paths understand that everything is perception. What you think is real is a product of your beliefs that determine how you look at things. Both paths believe that energy and intention can help you manifest anything.

Differences

The predominant difference between the two paths is how they predict the future. Historically, the shaman was relied upon to find the game for the next hunt and the next place the tribe to live. A shaman was a religious figure, a healer, a nurturer for the soul of the individual and the tribe. The Tantric took much responsibility for the tribe's spiritual health, if not physical health. Through Tantric ritual, the individual was initiated into the spiritual world and the adult world. As a representative of the Great Mother, the Tantric would energetically and physically bring young people into their own as a sexual/spiritual being, so that they could fully experience all that he was. Dance and sexuality were all part of the celebration of being a spiritual being. What is energy medicine and why is it becoming so popular? Energy medicine has been around for thousands of years, mostly in the form of spiritual or shamanic healing.

I think that just about sums it up. Science has convinced that if we can't measure it, it doesn't exist. Modern energy medicine workers, shamanic healers, know, without doubt, that is simply not true. From my point of view, energy medicine begins to bridge the gap between traditional forms of energy healing and new, more documented, forms. The roots are the same. The role of Spirit is the same. Once the shaman,(Paje) or the medicine woman or man, learns to tap into and read the energy world, he begins to form methods of healing and communicating with Spirit that work for her or him. Some folks are concerned that the new "shamans" are diluting the old traditions, when in fact, they are merely pushing the boundaries and redefining new paths to wholeness. The goal of energy medicine, as with many spirit-based traditions, is to help the individual be a whole person, not a collection of parts. Living fully, joyfully and healthfully, is an art and skill. It isn't just being healthy, but living beyond your human, culturally conditioned fears, where bliss and ecstasy reside.

The practice of Shamanism is nearly as old as human consciousness itself. Arising from a primary impulse toward *ecstacy*, the shaman seeks communion with all that is, and in the process adopts the role of mediator, counsel and healer to his or her community. Because he seeks union with nature in all its manifestations, he becomes conversant with the Natural Powers, and by following their guidance he is able to achieve feats denied to ordinary mortals. He is, however, bound to the rules of the cosmos, and as such, he or she is also entrusted with their safekeeping.

As steward of his environment, he must excel in discipline, and be at all times conscious of his position in the Universe. This privileged status does not come without hardship, and it is axiomatic that the initiate undergo ordeals of purification. These can take the form of vision quests, pilgrimages, or ritualized ordeals. Often, however, the initiate is thrust into his profession by the workings of the spirit world, and can inherit his mantle through spontaneous vision, near death experiences or a descent into sickness or insanity. Regardless of the manner in which this discovery of the self is effected, the initiate is now on the path toward mastery. Shamanic knowledge the world over recognizes that all of Life is Power, and it is the task of the shaman to become conversant with the purveyors of such Power.

In order to develop as a practitioner, the initiate must undergo periodic and sustained journeying into the various regions or realms of the World. In classic terms the World is divided into three realms. The initiate descends into the Lower World to seek an encounter with his own Shadow, and in this process becomes familiar not only with his limitations and personal deficiencies, but also with his own mortality, experiencing over and over his own death through painful dismemberment at the hand of the denizens of the Lower World. It is this experience which grants him the authority necessary to attempt an ascent to the Upper World, the world of Light and Vision. Carried by his familiar (usually, though not always, a spirit being of animal form) the shaman journeys through innumerable realms seeking guidance and wisdom as he travels. As he does, his sensory and perceptual centers undergo a rapid and dramatic transformation, for he is now able to see things denied other mortals. He becomes aware of the infinity of worlds contained within the Universe and of the immensity of the Mystery of Life.

As his ecstatic trance carries him further and further away from the world of ordinary concern, he also hears a new calling. It is the voices of his community, which clamors in suffering and in pain. Moved by the compassion which is now his hallmark, he initiates a return to the Middle World, the world of ordinary concern, where he is now empowered to act as mediator, counsel, and healer.

In order for the Initiate to explore the realms of Existence it is necessary to have a map or a cosmic diagram of the various regions of the world. This knowledge is usually ancestral, and is handed from master to initiate in proscribed, traditional ways. Often the process is arduous, as the master trains the initiate into the subtleties of his trade by constant test and privations, as it is necessary for the initiate to fully comprehend the multilayered nature of the teachings. Often these are encoded in Myth, and are therefore capable of interpretation at many levels. As the student progresses, his understanding of the deceptively simple story grows. All of shamanic knowledge is holographic in the sense that each part is so designed as to contain the whole. In this respect it attempts to mirror the world, in which all is connected and in which interdependence is fundamental for survival. Simultaneously, the apprentice is also being instructed by teachers from the unseen realms. From these two sources (the world of ordinary teachers of flesh and blood and those of other realms) the initiate begins to map his own way through the landscape of a new existence he did not even suspect could have existed, because he/she was inert in maya (illusory reality).

In its external form, the cosmic vision of the shaman consists in an understanding of the forces of nature in relation to the four fold division of the horizon. The geomagnetic forces of the globe are taken as a departure point to create a framework of relationships that enables the practitioner to manipulate the forces to his design. The world is therefore understood as consisting of the following relationships:

North is conceived as the area of Darkness, and is therefore associated with tectonic forces, Mother Earth, the Body, and with reality as a manifestation in Space and Time.

South is conceived as the area of Light, and as such is the vehicle for divine illumination, Spirit, Wind, and the Eternal. East is the rising point of the Sun and as such corresponds to the awakened Mind, and to the Force of Fire. West is the setting Sun, and as such it is harbinger of the Moon, as well as the Subconscious and the Emotional aspect of consciousness. Its force is Water. At the Center is the World Tree, the Central Pillar that supports the heavens and through which the shaman ascends or descends in his journeys through the Realms. The center is the Void, where physical resistance can be minimized, and achievement made harmonious and balanced. It is often referred to as the Navel of the World, because of its associations with gestation and rebirth. The center is also the vehicle for the Sacred Thunderbolt of Illumination, carried or delivered by the bird ally, often the eagle or the hummingbird. The Center is often associated with the rainbow, and can be embodied in the Drum. Its counterpart is the Forge, where the thunderclap of the mallet shapes the initiate into new forms and potentialities. In many Cultures the first shaman(Paje) is a smith, giver of measure and fire, and is therefore associated with Saturn, the God that measures the depths of the Universe. In addition to the four geomagnetic corners, archaic knowledge recognized the transverse axes of the solstices and equinoxes and used those markers for its description of time as an eternal return. These transverse axes were also seen mirrored in the heavens by the Milky Way, the road in the sky through which journeyed the souls of the dead and of the ancestors, traversing in and out of the Middle World through passages at points in the horizon where the constellations met the rising or setting sun during the winter and summer solstices. The shaman therefore conceives of the World as a four sided multidimensional structure, anchored at the "four corners" of the compass by "four pillars" which support the roof or "ridge pole" (also known as the tai chi among the Chinese). The Cosmos is often referred to as a house, or a tent, and spoken of as being "square" or "flat" not to imply a flat plane, but as a reference to the plane of the celestial equator. Archaic cultures also recognized the tilted plane of the ecliptic, the apparent path of the sun through the constellations, and referred to the relationship between the celestial equator and the ecliptic (set at an angle of approximately twenty-three degrees) as the "separation of the world parents." The myth of the "end of the world" so common throughout the world cultures is a reference to the transit of the key constellation of each world era through changing areas in the sky due to the precession of the equinoxes. This mythology implies a thorough understanding on the part of the ancient astronomer priests of the existence of the plane of the ecliptic at a very early stage in human history. The axis of rotation of the world around the "nail" star (Polaris in our age) is referred to variously as the "cosmic pillar" or World Mountain, or often as the World Tree or "ladder" which the shaman must climb in his ascent to the Upper World. It is evident from overwhelming evidence worldwide, that all shamanic cultures excelled at astronomy. In most myths of origin, the first shaman is either a smith who fashions the heavens or the one entrusted with the measurement of the skies. The shaman is therefore fully capable of mapping and traveling throughout the cosmos, because he has seen in vision and confirmed through his observation of the movement of the stars the multidimensional nature of the Cosmos.

This initial education into the structure and design of the Cosmos, however, must be later abandoned for a surrender to the very same forces the initiate once attempted to control. It is in this dialectic between longing (for union with the Cosmos), desire (for mastery and service), and surrender that the shaman finds mastery. Once mastery is achieved, the shaman becomes a hollow vessel for the mystical forces of Nature to act through, "no ego".

The shaman conceives of Reality as a vast web of interconnections, animated by the Sacred Power of the Divine. All that exists is alive and has spirit, and can therefore partake of the bounty as well as the suffering of the World. The web of power animates the Cosmos.

Anybody or anything is capable of exercising this power. It is therefore axiomatic that all things are worthy of respect and care. What we do to others will ultimately affect us through the myriad interconnections which unite us into one single holographic whole.

It is the task of the shaman to become aware of the Power in the World, for it is this power which is constantly at work, changing and transforming one thing into another. It speaks through its manifold manifestations, and can be encountered everywhere. Experience, therefore is not a burden to the shaman, but a crucible through which to understand the messages of power. It acts through us and through all that is.

The ordeals which the shaman endures as his or her vision is awakened are often painful,(most, when foresees the future) but the end result is a transformation of the individual from a profane entity into one that is sacred. To maintain this stature is arduous work, as the rules and norms of conduct of society and cosmos must be faithfully adhered to. Failure to do so creates great danger. The shaman, however, cannot turn back, as his life carries him or her on into deeper and deeper layers of the cosmic vision he is now embodying. It is at this stage that the shaman becomes healer and myth-maker as well.

For the master shaman, time and space have been suspended, as all times are subsumed into the "now" and all places into the "here." In every detail of his experience, the shaman sees miracles and finds new worlds revealed. It is this ecstatic vision which is his greatest legacy, for it points the way not toward that which is, but toward that which can be. The material gives way to the eternal, the base to the enlightened, and thus meaning is achieved.

Tantra

"Not to all and any should this hymn be revealed For be it made known to one who is unworthy, Then ill falls upon him. Therefore should it be carefully concealed."
Practices . . .

Sexual Ritual

Yamala-the Tantric Couple

The sexual practices of the *Kaula* school, also known as the *the secret ritual*, are based on the couple. They are performed with a so-called *external Sakti* (sexual partner) as opposed to the purely meditative practices which involve only one's own spiritual energies (the interior Sakti or Shakti).

Abhinavagupta gives a pretty radical definition of the Tantric couple, from the point of view of an illuminated master: "The couple (*yamala*) is consciousness itself, the unifying emission and the stable abode. It is the absolute, the noble cosmic bliss consisting of both Siva or Shiva and Shakti. It is the supreme secret of *Kula*; neither quiescent nor emergent, it is the flowing font of both quiescence and emergence." Tantra Loka. (*Loka* is a Sanskrit word for "world").

Thus the ultimate form of the Tantric couple is identical to the Shiva Shakti couple (balance between male and female sexual energy to enhance kundalini). The two lovers are not merely mimicking the Divine Couple, but becoming one with it, and respectively with one another. This state combines both the dynamic and the static aspects of the Divine.

The role of the sexual *Kaula* ritual is to unite the couple yogini (initiated woman) and siddha (initiated man) and induce one in the other a state of permanent awakening This achievement made possible by the intensity of their love. The right bundle of entheogens enhance that state of awareness (*SEE JABABA*) *and achieve the soma state of spiritual awareness.*

First the mental limitations will fall and the force centers will harmonize their energies. In their exalted state, the two become absorbed into consciousness. Becoming united on all the levels, physical, astral, mental and even in their consciousness, they reconstitute the supreme couple of Shiva and Shakti.

The *Kaula* sacrifice is reserved for the few, the elites, who can maintain a state of *Bhairava* (spiritual illumination) while being engaged in the sexual union. Other couples, even if they reproduce the ritual to the letter (as perceived from outside), if they do not attain the *Bhairava* consciousness, are merely making love.

This path to spiritual accomplishment is considered fast but very difficult. Making use of the enormous forces sleeping inside human sexual potential, the *secret ritual* accelerates the evolution, but also the risk of failure thus the need for it to remain a secret.(handling the right tools wisely easy the path!!! "entheogen") Otherwise we'd have both people failing in their spiritual endeavors (on its account), and a lot of misconception distorting the purpose of this ritual. As any ritual, it lives in the energies accumulated through repetition, over many years allowing incomplete or distorted applications would be detrimental to its efficacy.

Called initiation by the mouth of the yogini (*yoginīvaktra*), it is a method by which the adept unites with a purified *yoginī* (advanced female practitioner) and receives the unique experience of the illuminated consciousness directly from her. He is to see her as both his lover and guru. Such practices allow for the transmission of the initiation first from the guru to his female disciples, and then from them to the male disciples, in the end closing the circle.

Sexual Sounds

Focusing on lovemaking sounds (*HĀ-HĀ*) of the woman leads to the "undivided level."

Sexual Fluids

The sexual fluids are considered to be endowed with the powers of consciousness. The fluids are called "kula."
The three forms of emission:
The energy generated during the Tantric sexual act is considered a form of *subtle emission*, while the act of ejaculation is considered a form of *physical emission*. Depending on the orientation of one's consciousness, introverted or extroverted, emission can be of two kinds:
Santa is the rested form of emission, when the focus is resting just on the self. It is associated with a state of transcendence.
Udita is the risen form of emission where the focus is resting on the other (the partner in love). This emission is associated to the state of immanence.
Santodita—beyond *udita* and *santa*—is the uniting form, cause of both santa and *udita* emissions. *Santodita* is described as universal bliss (*cidananda* or *jagadananda*), undivided consciousness and *kaula*.

Abhinavagupta describes this state as the outflow of the pulsation of Shiva and Shakti, undivided and complete.

(Abhinavagupta, was born in the Valley of Kashmir in a family of scholars and mystics and studied all the schools of philosophy and art of his time under the guidance of many teachers and gurus, a genius of his time).

"These two aspects, passive [santa] and active [udita]," explains Abhinava, "arise at the same time in the power and its possessor. The active passes from one domain to the other; the passive is confined within the self [the essential nature of both]. But even so, in reality, each of them form a couple [yamala]. Hence, the emergent is the quiescent."

Santodita, quiescence, and emergence

1: *nijananda*—the state of self repose
2: *nirananda*—nonbliss
3: *parananda*—satiation of the senses; pleasure found in external objects, but without the sense of AHAM "self" Associated to *udyoga* (creative outburst)
4: *brahmananda*—attention is drawn toward consciousness; a sense of wonder Associated to *avabhasa* (manifestation)
5: *mahananda*—a stage of *bliss* where one is intensely focused on his loved one; passionate, mutual absorption; heightened consciousness—Associated to *carvana* (devouring)
6: *cidananda*—the couple loses all sense of differentiation; complete union; reaching the pinnacle of consciousness; the united form of emission Associated to *visranti* (repose)
7: *jagadananda*—universal bliss, expansiveness; the whole world is seen as coming from them and destined to them;

becoming the supreme Kaula, transcending emanation and resorption

Mantric Practice

Mantric meditation is the most common form of Tantric practice. In the *Kaula* system, this practice is associated especially with the group of phonemes. The fifty phonemes (*varna*) of the Sanskrit alphabet are used as mantras denoting various aspects of consciousness (*cit*) and energy (*sakti*). The group (*kula*) of Sanskrit phonemes form a complete description of reality, from the lowest (*earth*) to the highest (*Siva* consciousness) level. The ritual "setting out" of the phonemes imitate the emanation of the cosmos from the supreme consciousness of Siva. In another ritual, the phonemes are identified with specific zones of the body through the practice of *nyasa*, infusing the body with spiritual energy. This mystical state of culminates in the *kaula* of the body and such a being is known as a siddha (accomplished one). The adept attains a form of bodily enlightenment where, through the power of mantras, one comes to recognize the divinities within the body. Initiation in the mantric practice is based on a transfer of power and the link (lineage) of the heart. Thus, simple knowledge of the word or phoneme is not useful in itself, as it does not have efficiency, unless the disciple received his initiation from an authentic master. Even if the concept of mantra is primarily related to shakti, it is necessary to remember that Sakti and Siva are always united. Thus, the supreme mantra, *paravak,* is equated to I-consciousness of the Lord·

A *mantra* is a religious syllable or poem, typically from the *Sanskrit* language. Their use varies according to the school and philosophy associated with the mantra. They are primarily used as spiritual conduits, words and vibrations that instill one pointed concentration(focus) in the devotee. Other purposes have included religious ceremonies to accumulate wealth, avoid danger, or eliminate enemies. Mantras originated in *India* with *Vedic Hinduism* and were later adopted by Buddhists and Jains, now popular in various modern forms of spiritual practice which are loosely based on practices of these *Eastern religions*.

The word "*mantra*" is a Sanskrit word consisting of the root *man*—"manas or mind" and the suffix-*tra* meaning, tool, hence a literal translation would be "mind tool." Mantras are interpreted to be effective as sound (vibration), to the effect that great emphasis is put on correct pronunciation (resulting in an early development of a science of phonetics in India). They are intended to deliver the mind from illusion and material inclinations. Chanting is the process of repeating a mantra. The most basic mantra is *Om/Aum*, which in Hinduism is known as the "pranava mantra," the source of all mantras. The philosophy behind this is the Hindu idea of namarupa (name form), which supposes that all things, ideas or entities in existence, within the phenomenological cosmos, have name and form of some sort. The most basic name and form is the primordial vibration of Aum, as it is the first manifested namarupa of Brahman the unmanifested reality/unreality. Essentially, before existence and beyond existence is only One reality, Brahman, and the first manifestation of Brahman in existence is Aum. For this reason, *Aum is considered to be the most fundamental and powerful mantra,* and thus is prefixed and suffixed to all Hindu prayers. While some mantras may invoke individual *Gods* or principles, the most fundamental mantras, like

Aum, the Shanti Mantra, the Gayatri Mantra, and others all ultimately focus on the One reality.

In the Hindu Tantras the universe is sound. The supreme (para) brings forth existence through the Word (Shabda). Creation consists of vibrations at various frequencies and amplitudes giving rise to the phenomena of the world. The purest vibrations are the varna, the imperishable letters which are revealed to us, imperfectly as the audible sounds and visible forms.(Varna system of Brahminical society)

Aum is one of the most popular chants in India. if done properly, it can be a door to silence. Below is a technique, which I learned, from Osho teachings.

A caution from Osho: A mantra has to be chanted and then dropped. A mantra is complete only when you can drop it. Do not cling to it! the teachings presented here does came from him, learned from his discourses and his teachings.

How to chant the Aum mantra. Osho's teachings, delivered through his discourses, were not presented in an academic setting, but interspersed with jokes and delivered with a rhetoric that many found spell binding. The emphasis was not static but changed over time: Osho reveled in paradox and contradiction, making his work difficult to summarize. He delighted in engaging in behavior that seemed entirely at odds with traditional images of enlightened individuals; his early lectures in particular were famous for their humor and their refusal to take anything seriously. All such behavior, however capricious and difficult to accept, was explained as a technique for transformation "to push people" beyond the mind.

He spoke on major spiritual traditions including Jainism, Hinduism, Hassidism, Tantrism, Taoism, Christianity, Buddhism, on a variety of

Eastern and Western *mystics* and on sacred scriptures such as the Upanishads and the Guru Granth Sahib.

First stage, sit down relaxed, either in a temple or in your room and repeat AUM as loudly as possible, for one hour. Use the whole body to repeat it, as if thousands of people are listening to you without a microphone, and you have to be very loud so that the whole body trembles, shakes with it. Let the body be saturated with the sound of Aum.

For almost three months, you should not bother about anything else, and only practice this first stage. The first stage is very important because it gives the foundation.

Second Stage

After three months, when you feel your body is completely saturated, when you can feel deep down inside you that the word has entered into the body cells, as if your whole body can repeat it; then you are ready for the second step. The second step is to close your mouth and repeat and chant the word "Aum mentally." The throat, the tongue, the lips, everything should be closed, the whole body locked, and this chanting should only be in the mind but as loudly as possible: with the same loudness you were using with the body. Now allow the mind too to be saturated with Aum.

Third stage

When the mind feels saturated . . . it is just like eating: you feel full, when it is enough; so also the mind will feel full when it is enough. Then starts the third step. Neither the body has to be used nor the mind has to be used at this stage. Just listen, and you will hear a sound coming to you from your own heart of hearts. The Aum will be there inside you, as if somebody else is chanting; and you are just the listener.

This is the completion of the chant mantra.

A mystical system

Kaula is an esoteric system based on complex Tantric symbolism, obscure to rational analysis, but rather suited for direct practical experience. In order to grasp it, one needs to be initiated, a process which implies a mystic transfer of energy (descent of the sakti) that will *open the disciple's heart* and reveal the truth. The core of mystical practices is considered to be an inner teaching that form the basis and origin of the sophisticated philosophical systems of [Kashmir Shaivism] even if they might seem more primitive at first glance

Kaula puts extreme emphasis on experiential replication

Intuitive revelation

The mere knowledge of the Kashmir Shaivism methods of attaining shiva are considered enough to procure liberation by a process of intuition (*prathiba*) Spiritual intuition is described as a process of descent of the Shakti transmitting a form of *knowledge beyond discursive thinking.*

While the more philosophical doctrines of Kashmir Shaivism form the "outer teachings," Kaula represents the "inner teachings," esoterical aspects aimed at *the attainment of enlightenment.*

Rudra Yamala Tantra, Kularnava Tantra, Svaccanda Tantra, Netra Tantra, Tantraraja Tantra, the Tantraloka.

From an exterior/interior point of view, *Kaulika-siddhi* can be seen as both extroverted and introverted. Its extroverted aspect is that of instrument of perception (the whole body-mind complex being itself is a *Kula*, thus, having *Kaulika* shakti as its unifier). On the other side, the introverted aspect of *Kaulika-siddhi* is that of pure I-consciousness, the substrate of all the objective and subjective life.

If *Kula* is the limited consciousness, *Akula* is the absolute Consciousness (parasamvit), the unsurpassed reality (*anuttara*) and uncreated light (*Prakasa*). Limited consciousness is seen as a mere external object compared to the supreme consciousness *Cit*, which can never be an object of contemplation itself as it is the pinnacle of the subjectivity.

Kauliki (Shakti) is the energy of *Akula* (Shiva), identical to self awareness (*Vimarsa*), the sleeping bodily energy (*Kundalini*), the force of emission (*Visarga*), beatitude of the Siva-Sakti union (*Ananda*). Thus under various names there is only one force.

Kauliki acts as a perfect mirror, reflecting in it both the supreme (*Akula*) and the manifested (*Kula*), "mirror" that is identical to the cosmic beatitude (*ananda*)

Kauliki (shakti, *ananda*) is thus said to be the supreme energy, containing all possibilities, full of all qualities, pervading everything from the absolute down to the material plane and reflecting everything in itself as mere aspects. "Pervading everything "is another way of saying "reflecting everything in itself." The idea here is that wherever there is manifestation or even in the absolute itself, the *Kauliki* energy is the ubiquitous substrate.

Kauliki pervades at various levels—supreme, mental, physical, social consciousness—is all pervading, true nature.

Kauliki is an all-pervading energy, nothing being outside its realm. The notion of containing everything manifested in itself is described sometimes as "reflecting "everything in itself like a mirror. The levels which are pervaded (reflected) in *Kauliki* seem to be arranged on a sliding scale, from the largest to the smallest unit of manifestation. In order, from interior to exterior, they are:

The absolute, denoted also as:
  anuttara–unsurpassable
  akula–beyond objectivity
  Shiva–The Lord
  Cit–supreme consciousness
  Prakasa–uncreated light

The supreme energy–also known as:
  Vimarsa–power to reflect
  Visarga–power to emit the creation (universe)
  Shakti–the divine energy
  Kundalini–the coiled divine energy, sleeping inside
      the body
  Ananda–supreme bliss

The limited subjects (mental level)
   The mental group (*Kula*) being made of the five senses, sensorial mental, ego and intellect

The exterior objects (material level)
   The physical body—a *Kula* of the organs and instruments of the body
   External objects—a *Kula* of material objects that rely on the first five tattvas (the thirty-six tattvas), from prithivi to akasa

The spiritual family (social level)
   A group based on brotherly love, common spiritual aims and openness, led by a master who has revealed his supeme self, Atman.

Kaula refers to *Kula* (Shakti), *Akula* (Shiva) and their manifestations, all of which form reality. *Kaula* is knowledge in its three aspects of knower, known and knowing

Liberation (*moksa*) is nothing else than the revelation of one's nature, and one's nature is simply consciousness of the self.

Initiation does not give what is not already known, but rather cuts bonds which might hinder a person from self recognition

The body-union of yoni and lingam

The subtle breath (unification of prana and apana)

Consciousness (unification of the subject and object, all the objects of the senses are offered as sacrifice to consciousness); the fire of consciousness devours everything that is dual

The adept of *Kaulism* cultivates either Anavopaya or Shambhavopaya

The Kaula ritual is accomplished in thought, word or action, in worldly activities, in relation to a woman, in couple, in the body, breath and thought

The effortless method—Sambhavopaya—direct and immediate entry in nirvikalpa

Udyoga, avabhasa, carvana and *visranti* are the four steps of the *Krama* system.

Perineum

The portion of the body in the pelvis occupied by urogenital passages and the rectum, bounded in front by the pubic arch, in the back by the coccyx, and laterally by part of the hipbone. The region between the scrotum and the anus in males, and between the posterior vulva junction and the anus in females, this secretive key point is used in more advanced tantric practices, to hold "libido" triggering, multiple orgasms, and halting physical ejaculation.

God Spot and Clitoris

The Grafenberg spot or G-spot or God spot is a small spot in the genital area of women behind the pubic bone and surrounding the urethra. G-spot is a bundle of nerves within the vaginal canal that often produces pleasurable sensations when stimulated. It is usually located about halfway between the back of the pubic bone and the front of the cervix, along the course of the urethra and near the neck of the bladder, where it connects with the urethra. G-spot is a spongy ridged area inside the vagina. Stimulating the G-spot can produce *sexual pleasure to the extreme level,* this is the key to eliminate blocks of stress and help find balance between Ida and Pingala. The clitoris is a small budlike formation situated at the top of the inner vaginal lips. Normally, it is hidden under a small hood of skin, but expands when sexually aroused. Most women can attain orgasm by means of gentle massage of the clitoral area. Biologically, it is directly equivalent to the male penis. You've probably spent a considerable amount of time studying the female G-spot, how to find it, how to stimulate it, and how to turn a woman into putty with a G-spot orgasm. What most men are far less familiar with is their own male G-spot. That's right; some of you may be surprised to learn that the prostate is, essentially, the male equivalent of a woman's G-spot. This is the key to release blocks of accumulated stress and also helping clean our chakras promoting some kind of helicoidally motion in it, more we feed our chakras with sexual energy better they functioning. Only than our work can run smoothly, this is imperative to send the sexual energy to our heads.

Sakti the ultimate Shakti, the ultimate feminine power.

Shakti, meaning sacred *force*, *power*, or *energy*, is the Hindu concept or personification of the divine In traditional Shiva associated Shaktism, Shaktism regards Devi ("the Goddess") as the Supreme Brahman itself, the "one without a second," with all other forms of divinity, female or male, considered to be merely her diverse manifestations. In the details of its philosophy and practice, Shaktism resembles Saivism. However, *Shaktas (Sanskrit: Sakta)*, practitioners of Shaktism, focus most or all worship on Shakti, as the dynamic feminine aspect of the Supreme Divine. Shiva, the masculine aspect of divinity, is considered solely transcendent, and Shiva's worship is generally relegated to an auxiliary role. In Vaishnavism, like Shiva associated Shaktism, Shakti embodies the active feminine energy and power of male supreme deity Vishnu in Vaishnavism. Vishnu's female counterpart is called Lakshmi. However, in Srivaishnavism, a school of Vaishnavism, Lakshmi or Sri does not play any particular part in the creative function of the Lord, because Prakriti is the manifest aspect of the Lord. In Srivaishnavism, Vishnu alone is the great creator, although Sri is coeval with him. As Vishnu is the Father who stands for absolute justice, Sri is the Mother of the universe and is considered to be important element in the redemption of mankind, and is the interceder with Vishnu on behalf of spiritual seekers.

"Lord Krishna, among many others qualities, is the intellectual manifestation of the sexual energy."

Goithyja

> *"Kundalini.* The kundalini resides in the sacrum bone in three and a half coils and has been described as a residual power of pure desire *libidinal* force or Shakti, lies coiled at the base of the spine in male and females as one!"

Consciousness and Intention

We are ready as a species to looker deeper than just the surface of matter. Indeed, peering deeply into and beyond matter through *quantum physics*, we see that the hard stuff *we perceive as matter* does not exist. Instead we are presented with a dance of energy that is beyond rational explanation. More fascinating is research into how the brain assembles our world. Based on how the brain processes signals in the dream state and waking consciousness we cannot conclusively prove that the world before us exists. It is self evident that awareness of consciousness exists. We can prove consciousness exists through the adage "I think. Therefore I am" (self, ego). Rather than attempting to understand outer mechanics through physics *we should be launching expeditions into the realms of consciousness.* The human heart is able to make connections to people, places, and things regardless of our perceived distances of space or time. The domain of the heart allows us to make connections that are as well, and sometimes more real, than physical locality. If you are willing to approach through this book with sincerity then you can receive many of the same energetic initiations as those who use this as a guidebook to reach higher levels of consciousness, It was with these perspectives in mind and accompanied by a great sense of purpose that this book was undertaken. I had to return from my shamanic trips, prepared to write the book. I was not really clear at that time what the content of my first book was to be. But this book you are reading now is the result of a serious of fortuitous events highlighted by the use of entheogenic substances in the ritualistic sacramental way. That was my call to right this book to pass this knowledge too as many people as I can, to demonstrates to people, harmony with the many energies and sublime forces who does involve around us. Indeed the perspective is that we live on the skin of and feed from the breast of Mother Earth and we are more deep connected with the universe than we thought of it. The Sun Father watches overhead providing warmth and energy for everything we need to grow. The rain blesses us with water for drinking, bathing, irrigation, and play. We look to the hummingbird as a sign of the joy of spirit. This perspective is achieved when we first realize our place in this grand family of life. This is a vignette into the earthy yet spiritual radiance of the people around the world and indeed much of South America where we can still find a reach of entheogenic herbs, fungi, and psychedelic toads among others.

There are many similarities between western civilization and more native, other solar cultures. Like Ancient Egypt the spiritual harmonization of the Inka attunes itself both to terrestrial and solar consciousness. The Andean psyche in South America resembles most of the ancient civilizations on earth associates various animal archetypes with the internal progress on the spiritual path. In the shamanic culture three animals typify the three worlds. The serpent represents the lower world. The puma represents our middle world. The condor represents the upper world. These power animals also represent mastery over that world. Any developing spiritual culture and individual persona must first deal with the energies at the level of the serpent. The serpent's expression of the divine is not as much limited as it is foundational. In another deep Jungian aspect the serpent symbolizes our undulating DNA. Shamans who drink the Amazonian ayahuasca psychedelic tea report the serpent as a common motif in their experiences. The ayahuasca vine itself is shaped like a serpent. The serpent has also been recognized by the indigenous people to symbolize the untransformed ego.

The serpent is consciousness at the level that crawls upon the ground. Viewed from this aspect a serpentine consciousness is reactive and has not achieved mastery over self. Once we learn both our strengths and shortcomings we usually question our place in the world. This inner reorientation usually comes in the form of a mid life crisis, dark night of the soul, or other spiritual emergence. At this point we typically commit ourselves to the spiritual path. A process of inner refinement is often accompanied metaphysically by activation of the *kundalini* life energy that also follows the serpent metaphor. When our personal transformation has begun we learn how to use the basic serpent level energies to empower our life's path. Often we find that when the spiritual life has begun in earnest then we immediately want to take up our wings and fly like birds or angels. A sense of breaking free from the gravity of mundane life unlocks our imagination and opens immense possibilities for personal growth. Our inner spirit often compels us to undertake spiritual pilgrimage to the ocean or to the mountains. Our hearts long to more fully manifest a breaking free of the constraints of life as we have known it and to seek reunification with the spiritual essence of all things. In the shamanic worldview this is the realm of the Condor or Horus, who was the ancient Egyptian sky god who was usually depicted as a falcon. The Condor soars high above the earth communing with the Creator of life. To the indigenous people of South America this union of serpent wisdom and life force combined with the wings of flight to become respective interpretations of the same spiritual forces of Quetzalcoatl. (Pinchbeck talks about that in his book *The Return of Quetzalcoatl*, a highly recommended book to read.) Quetzalcoatl is the rainbow colored flying serpent. The spiritually refined personality finds the way to harness the energies and experiences of living upon the earth in order to take flight to the higher spiritual domains. Today we are witnesses to the return of Quetzalcoatl both individually and collectively. By the way, something pop up on my mind!, I do believe in reality the true story of the bible concerning Adam and Eve and the serpent of knowledge is just the hundalini power being tempted by Eve's "pussy" represented by the apple, cut in half an apple, and what do you see sick minded guy? so ? did you get the picture ? another crooked tale from the bible, which until this days elude lots of people, trapped in "maya", the idea is keep the sexual energy and not dissipate it. To become more enlightened, to the head we go! I do not know if the Roman catholic church is trying to hide the truth or if they are just trapped in "maya" like most people.

The sacred mythic tones of the past are being sounded again in our time. In the shamanic spiritual domain it is the puma that resides in and represents this middle world that we live in. Egyptian symbols like the sphinx and Sekhmet convey the power of the divine feminine to empower human life. The goal of the human spiritual life is to be a living and breathing human expression of the divine being with balance between both realities. It is this transformed personality that the puma represents. To become a puma you must observe the reactive ego "self" and gain mastery over it. Reforming the ego is an act of love, not just power. It takes the courage of the puma to see the shortcomings of self and others and still walk with an open heart. *Dissolve our egos is not easy task!,* In a certain sense the puma is another way to view Quetzalcoatl the winged serpent. The earth body joins with the winged inspiration of the heavens to form a divine being that walks upon the earth. This refined puma person is called a Puma Runa. The repeated iconography of the puma in shamanism emphasizes the importance of living as a divine lion hearted human being. It is the puma that integrates the Mother Earth, Sun Father, all things, into the heart of the truly divine human. Unveiling is a spiritual development that the puma person can stand as a divine solar initiate. Just as the sphinx that stands next to the pyramids in Egypt, the puma person stands on the earth being astounded daily of the presence of the divine solar being as their self. The Buddha and the Christ are said to take the middle way. The shamans say the same thing. To live as a divine puma person on the earth is to balance all the energies of the universe while walking in the flesh. There is a divine mission to be accomplished by those who walk in this manner. These beings are the puma people, the modern shamans within. All spiritual lineages encode the subtle bodies of their initiates with specific information related to the function of that group. The codes of light committed to the shamanic lineage are expressed through sacramental knowledge and sacred entheogenic and Tantric rituals. The same storehouses of shamanic knowledge and wisdom are sitting now right in front us. Places like the rain forest resonate with archaic consciousness in sublime and active ways as containers to hold cosmic energy and the spiritual energy of the shamans. Places that have additionally been engineered as premier sacred living machines by God possess the added benefit of having been formed as explicit conductors of the highest spiritual energies known. It is not an exaggeration to say that *when walking through the rain forest in South America, you are walking in the footsteps and within the most primitive and beautiful of God's creation*—conscious awareness who plugs you into the same divine informational matrix that exists beyond time and space. If you walk under the effects of the right bundle of entheogens with awareness, you can have a very deep experience at many levels. But you will get more out of your experience if you use both your mind and your heart and tune into the information that is there. It is one thing to undertake a trip (deep into the forest, you feel your lungs with the ethereal pranic energy like no other place on earth) the cure is contagious. It is a completely different experience if you travel as a spiritual pilgrim expecting that your trip will have a significant outcome from the very beginning. This is the key to experience with entheogens with the guidance of a knowledgeable mystic like Goithyja the neophyte partake with the true meaning in dealing with entheogenic substances (awareness of God within).

In the Hindu religion, the movements of the expansion and contraction of the universe are viewed as the inhalation and exhalation of Brahma. *Higher spirituality tends toward a unification that is beyond the dualities of light and dark, good and evil, yin and yang.* When discussing these periods, it is important not to apply our cultural filters to these periods. Instead of alternating periods of absolute light and darkness, view these periods as phases of the moon. These periods are the dance of revelation and integration, of expansion and concentration. In the periods of "light," there is new spiritual information that propels consciousness forward. In the periods of "darkness," there is a period of integration. This cyclic alternation mirrors the change of the four seasons. The light of springtime brings growth that matures over the summer. From the growth of summer, the seeds of autumn are sown, which rest below the soil during the winter. In the West, the challenge for us is that our culture has removed us from the normal relationships with the earth that our passage through these time cycles produces unintended side effects. These side effects are most evident in the integrative or dark periods. During an integrative dark cycle, earth-based cultures are generally venturing inward and concretizing the wisdom of the previous light cycle through art, music, and mythology. Because our material civilization is not standing in a correct relationship with the earth, there is a shadow aspect of ourselves not properly aligned or expressed during the dark phases. When our culture enters a dark period of the time cycle, we tend toward the lower drives of fear and warfare. The isolation we find ourselves in comes from cutting off our recognition of or encounter with the irrational and mysterious forces of nature. For instance, how many adolescents today reaffirm their relationship to the earth and the community by undergoing rites of passage? Increasingly in Western, nineteen—or twenty-year-olds, especially young men, create their own psychic transitions that appear to be temporary psychosis. Who in our culture can tell these young people that they are undergoing a psychic reorientation rather than just having an acute chemical imbalance to be treated Invasively with foreign chemicals? At a time these young people most need ceremony and community support we drug them and temporarily commit them to mental wards. The psychic and sacred do not exist easily within the clinical and larger scientific nomenclature. *Due to our fragmentation and separation from the sacred* in Western society the least desirable behaviors tend to be exhibited during the time cycle dark phases. In written history these recurring phases tend to be times of prolific or global strife, warfare, and ignorance. But these side effects are not a function of the time cycles but of our disintegrated cultural psyche. So keep in mind as we talk about the time cycles that the dark periods are not inherently bad. It is our culture that reacts badly within them. The methods and ways of Western civilization are under scrutiny and many old things that do not work are being set aside. Environmentalism, New Age, Conscious Living, Alternative, are all energized by what seems to be a world that is speeding up. *We are clearly, from all sides and indicators, in a time of great, if not immense change.* Accompanying this undercurrent is a great sense of uncertainty and often fear. We have been taught to look for the solutions from somewhere, anywhere, outside of ourselves. If only the wise ones, the great leaders and healers of old, were here to help us make it through. The people who are going to make it through this transition are already here. Instead of looking outside for the answers maybe we need to look inside. The allies we have in the trek of life and wisdom are known to us.

Trust in the beauty of the inner self. *Trust in the loving arms of shamanic path.* Trust in the earth, air, water, fire, and sun. Our helpers are forces and angels of light and *love*. Yet to really make this all happen, a transition to a world of wisdom and beauty, it takes you and me. The ability, in our time, for someone from Amsterdam or Perth or Tokyo, to be able to travel to a place like *the Amazon rain forest is significant.* You can pay for special tours to receive some initiations. But walking around, is an initiation in its own right. The consciousness of the shamanic path again awakens. You can associate this with the ending of the Pachacuti (most archaeologists now believe that the famous Inca site of Machu Picchu was built as an estate for Pachacuti), of darkness in the period from 1992-2012 CE. There is harmonic convergence and harmonic concordance. You have cosmic emissions from the center of the galaxy and magnetic gravity waves acting as metaphysical sources of transformation inspiration. We are in a universe far stranger and more alive in ways that science is only beginning to allow into their paradigms. At a deeper level what is really happening is a process of self-reflexive unfolding as part of a universal consciousness.

Some North American Indian prophesies pointed to the age and culture of the 1960s. These predictions stated that the children of the Europeans would seek an alternative to what their fathers told them and begin to seek the wisdom of the aboriginal elders. Still other messengers say that the souls Inkarnating now are from higher bands of consciousness. But in the end what matters is the experience itself, the rest is just a bunch of blah, blah, blah. By the sacramental use of shamanic entheogens with the help of ancient Tantric knowledge we can achieve higher levels of consciousness and prepare ourselves to the outcome, soon to unfold, over planet earth, the purification process. So be brave and prepare your body, mind and soul and have a nice trip back home, this is my best wishes as shaman and mystic to all of us. I do hope the knowledge in this book and in many others like this one can give you a glimpse to the entheogenic path starting with *ayahuasca glimpse!, I* would like to apologize to put too much emphasis in some topics, and if I did offend anyone, I do apologize; also, I have had no intentions to offend any dweller of our Mother Earth. Be in peace and love.

CHAPTER 9

Preparation

1. What entheogen would you like to try? Have had experience with? Do you have enough of it?

2. The place you are willing to have the sacrament is clean? There is no distractions?

3. The place must be like a Ashram (An ashram would typically, but not always, the ideal is be located far away from, human habitation, in forests, amid refreshing natural surroundings conducive to spiritual instruction and meditation. The residents of an ashram regularly performed spiritual and physical exercises, such as the various forms of Yoga. location, location, location have you ever heard that?

4. Clean it up, to engage into deep meditation states, without interruption of any kind.

5. No weapons of any kind or knifes on the place.

6. Empty stomach and intestine * (the whole digestive system must be clean)

7. Mind set, pure and clear spiritual thoughts only with only the best thoughts passing through your mind, this attitude can avoid the so-called bad trips.

8. Engage in Pranayama (Of these meanings, the concept of "vital air" is used by Bhattacharyya to describe the concept as used in Sanskrit texts dealing with pranayama. "prana" as "spirit energy." Its most subtle material form is the breath, but is also to be found in blood, and its most concentrated form is *semen in men and vaginal fluid in women*. Practice pranayama every day for fifteen minutes as form of meditation and also before taking any entheogenic solution.

9. Be prepared to meditate naked or with light white clothes never ever use dark ones

10. If do you have cats, dogs, birds "pets of any kind "keep them in a safe comfortable distance so, you can do your business without distractions

11. No phones or machines which suddenly can make noise

12. If you are religious make a prayer before taking the sacramental entheogenic portion, start with low doses always increasing in steps.

13. Having a friend (sitter) in a safe distance sometimes can help to keep novices calm.

14. Remember weak doses weak experiences but, even though, start always with small doses

15. If you do, have the opportunity to take the sacrament in a farm far away from the city surrounded by trees, is the best, because the environment is rich in prana.

16. I must put emphasis on this, keep always positive thoughts in your mind, clean mind clean experience, most of the time the so-called bad trips as mentioned before, is triggered by a duty digestive system including manly the liver (if is not clean), if the environment is peaceful, and clean most of the time the neophyte can have great spiritual experience.

17. Very important, guide your experience focusing in spiritual awareness, why I talk a lot about the Vedas, because can help guide you through, a spiritual path, this is the key to have a mystical religious experience

18. Forget materialistic things only have in your mind spiritual thoughts.

19. Using songs, meditative ones, can help send you strait to a more refined spiritual realm of learning, this is, what a shamanic guidance does provide, using songs and having, spiritual thoughts, sometimes dancing can help a lot.

20. The bad trip is only in the duty minds of those who experience the so-called bad trips, so keep your mind clean of bad thoughts.

21. Everything is created by the environment and your thoughts how clean your body is inside and out? and manly how clean your mind is ?

22. Try to rubbing your body with essential oil of camphor not the crude oil who is very powerful and can poison your skin but just the essential oil, use small amounts in your for head, chest and feet the feet are very important. This does help calm down your mind.

23. If in any way, you somehow get scared and you don't have a partner in hand to practice with ritualistic massages of the Tantra path, try to do it, with yourself enhancing the libido, this helps regain control over the experience.

24. The libido, avoiding ejaculation is the key to relaxation, using this technique you would avoid getting scared, if you have a reliable and dependable partner, the balance between two bodies is the best, yin and yang, male and female. The mystical experience or so-called soma state is achieved by keeping the libido as long as you can using the right entheogenic sacrament, do not forget the libido is the key to reach mystical awareness, but hold as long as you can, do not ejaculate, the ejaculation is only tolerated in the end of the ritual, applied mainly on novices, more, experienced psychonauts can hold

for a whole month such energy. As long you hold the libido without ejaculation, more and more you bring equilibrium to your chakras and nadis (In addition to the seven chakras of the subtle body, the Tantras have described a network of subtle channels known as Nadis. According to the Tantric treatise Shiva Samhita, there are fourteen principal nadis. Of these, Ida, Pingala and Sushumna are considered the most important. *Ida* is the left channel. Ida is white, feminine, cold, represents the moon and is associated with the river Ganges. Originating in Muladhara, Ida ends up in the left nostril. *Pingala* is the right channel. Pingala is red, masculine, hot, represents the sun and is associated with the river Yamuna. Originating in Muladhara, Pingala ends up in the right nostril. *Sushumna* is the central channel and is associated with the river Saraswati. Running up the body from just below Muladhara chakra to Sahasrara chakra at the crown of the head. *"pranayama"*

25. The objective is sending the sexual energy to your head, achieving, kundalini (Considered an advanced form of yoga and meditation, its purpose is to cultivate the creative spiritual potential of a human to uphold values, speak truth, and focus on the compassion and consciousness needed to serve and heal others)

26. This is the quantum leap to the whole experience, sending the sexual energy to your head and the opening of the third eye also, balancing the main nadis, Ida, Pingala, and sushumna nadis.

27. *Most people who take entheogens, only pay attention to the visual effects mind thoughts etc the most important thing is manipulate the most powerful energy of the universe and achieve Enlightenment.*

28. Soma state is direct correlated, with sexual energy and the right approach of the use of entheogenic substances, such knowledge was long hidden from main stream Westerners, but well know in the true shamanic and mystic way.

29. The mix of Tantra and entheogens, is the best of the best, because you will be dealing with Gods energy the sexual energy, so, flood your body cells with such energy. Your body is made with 100 percent, yes 100 percent, sexual energy and nobody can escape from that reality even the puritans all over the planet will one day end up knowing that. If they do deny that reality, they do deny life itself. Is like being denying themselves throughout their lives.

30. Set the right time and space for the ritual sacramental, find a place where no one unexpected will show up and where you feel at ease; also find the perfect time to completely get involved in the experience, without worrying about meetings, compromises, work or school (this can vary from four to ten or twenty-four hours, depending on the sacrament you are planning to use, sometimes even couple days)

33. Investigate the adequate dose for your specific herbal high and, if it's your first time attempting the psychotropic plant,

always start low ... extra low doses are better than a high dose of a psychedelic entheogen that you don't know how is going to affect your body, looks like I am repeating myself, but I do want to be sure you understood that quite well.

34. Get into the right *mind set*: it is important that you feel happy, excited and eager to live the experience, willing to change your perception and live something new.

   Never, ever, attempt an entheogenic experience with feelings of anger, depression, sadness or insecurity; you'll carry this emotional baggage with you and sabotage your trip. remember you are what you feed your mind soul and body.

35. Using legal, entheogens in the right countries, like Brazil, Peru, Portugal, etc, make the difference. "*Freedom* "in North America, people talk about freedom all the time, but, they really do experience that reality? or those are only wishes and thoughts into their minds?

36. Okay, time to dive into the experience ... play your favorite music (the style is important at this point), use meditation songs you can change later on, it as the psychotropic starts to work, do choice always peaceful songs).

37. Mentally review what it is that you want to get or experience with your chosen psychedelic entheogen and center yourself (close your eyes for a few minutes, take a few deep breaths,

relax..., to some entheogens like shrooms, best keep eyes opened...)

38. Take it in! eat, drink, or do whatever you have to do to get the entheogen into you. Remember, to take any entheogen you must have your body clean. *Do not forget taking a long bath or shower before starting the experience.* Also, you can take the entheogens naked or using light white clothes, never use dark colors (more refined and developed entities never approach duty environments, most of the time such beings help the neophyte throughout the experience), remember plants have their own consciousness so, go green avoid synthetics!

39. Be patient... the adventure will start any minute; sometimes it takes up to two hours to start peaking into the experience, so have music, calmly wait for it.

40. *BUM!*... This is it... now you're in the entheogens realm, let it work its magic into you.

41. *Don't analyze*, that comes later... let the experience flow naturally. Avoid using your intellect to make sense of what's happening; instead, confront everything that comes up during your experience, "surrender let the flow of the sacrament, carry you through the experience itself" they may be pleasant things, but they might as well be nightmares, it is a great opportunity to be face to face with your "self" and learn from it. if you do prepare your mind to the experience and have a

clean Environment with clean and fresh air, and throughout the experience you keep a positive attitude and you always keep positive thoughts in your mind, do you have a 96 percent chance to have a pleasurable and spiritual experience a true mystic one!, do not use entheogens in apartment buildings better use in houses (rural houses, far away from the storms of bad thoughts normally associate and found in the Unconscious mind of big cities, bad thoughts from great number of people leaving in those cities can trigger such situation). Also the right entheogen helps dissolve your ego so, naturally forcing the experience to run smoothly.

42. Maybe you'll want to have an audio recorder or pen and paper handy... some imagery or feelings will fade as the experience comes to an end.

43. If you start getting paranoid, scared or overwhelmed, always remember that it's just the entheogen inside you, it'll eventually go away... go to a quiet place, close your eyes, move around and take deep breaths, focusing on the air coming in and out... that usually helps to regain a little perspective. Remember before starting taking the entheogenic substance make pranayama for fifteen minutes, this does help balance your sexual energy. Accumulate also the sexual energy for one week before using the sacrament

44. Finally, have a place to crash near you... whenever you get tired or start coming down, go somewhere where you can lay down, close your eyes, and listen to some soothing music...

do not leave the place of meditation for twenty-four hours, do not operate any machinery during that period stay away from disturbance at any kind, you are in the transcendental states of awareness so, try to keep that for as long as you can, avoid conflicts.

45. This is the time to either fade away into the dream world, or meditate and think about what you have just experienced, until sleep naturally comes (it takes a couple of hours to come down from some entheogens, like LSD, and these last few hours of the trip can be a little harsh. It's a good idea to use that time and mind-set as a bridge or middle point to relate that divine experience to normal, everyday perception (this few hours are a point in between). Some people to do regain control faster, they do take guarana juice from true guarana (guaranine does not attack your nervous system like caffeine from coffee does, is not the same) do not use supplements and pills most of the time the labs do use caffeine from coffee not the true guaranine from guarana "I am from Brazil I do know guarana fruit quite well" or take the powerful Mahuang concentrated tea (*Ephedra sinica*) after the experience ends. "Go green go natural "do not take caffeine from coffee.

46. Take the next couple of days off from any mind altering substance . . . (ideally fifteen days)

47. *Now is the time to analyze what happened . . . Take some time to think about what you lived, what the magic plant has shown you, and how will the experience add up to your*

everyday life; every experience, done in the right set and setting can help you in becoming a better, brighter being.

48. I really encourage you to take the time to think about this, even if nothing pops into your mind at first what's the point of living a magical, divine experience if you forget all the realizations and insights you got as new situations, responsibilities and everyday matters keep coming up ?

49. Write down your thoughts and come back to them once in a while . . . Maybe in the future, when you want to re-experience the entheogen, you can also try different plants next time.

50. Intercalation (To insert among others) is also important experience with different entheogens every time you try a different one, more you learn from it. The plants of light have their own consciousness, "*unique ones.*"

"Having your period?" Avoid partake with entheogens, during that time (menstrual cycle),also be sure the entheogen will not generate an allergic reaction in your body.

"Let's talk little more, about kria yoga, kria, has a lot to do with tantra, entheogens and kundalini power."

Kriya Yoga is a set of yoga techniques that are the main discipline of Yogananda's meditation teachings. Kriya Yoga was passed down through Yogananda's guru lineage Mahavatar Babaji taught Kriya

Yoga to Lahiri Mahasaya, who taught it to his disciple Yukteswar, Yogananda's Guru. Because of ancient yogic injunctions, "the actual technique must be learned from a *Kriyaban* or *Kriya Yogi*," according to Yogananda. He gave a general description of Kriya Yoga in his Autobiography:

> "The Kriya Yogi mentally directs his life energy to revolve, upward and downward, around the six spinal centers (medullary, cervical, dorsal, lumbar, sacral, and coccygeal plexuses) which correspond to the twelve astral signs of the zodiac, the symbolic Cosmic Man. One-half minute of revolution of energy around the sensitive spinal cord of man effects subtle progress in his evolution; *that half minute of Kriya equals one year of natural spiritual unfoldment.*"

Balance and Good Humor (Mood)

At an early period, Ayurveda adopted the physics of the five elements (*Devanagari*); Prthvi (earth); Jala (water); Agni (fire); Vayu (air); and Akasa (Sky)—that compose the universe, including the human body. *Chyle* or plasma (called rasa dhatu*)*, blood (rakta dhatu*)*, flesh (mamsa dhatu*)*, fat (medha dhatu*)*, bone (asthi dhatu*)*, marrow (majja dhatu), and semen or female reproductive tissue (*sukra* dhatu*)* are held to be the seven primary constituent elements—*saptadhatu* (Devanagari*)* of the body. Ayurvedic literature deals elaborately with measures of healthful living during the entire span of life and its various phases. Ayurveda stresses a balance of three elemental energies or humors: Vayuvata (air and space—wind*)*, pitta (fire and water—bile*)* and kapha (water and earth—phlegm*)*.

According to ayurvedic medical theory, these three substances—dosas—are important for health, because when they exist in equal quantities, the body will be healthy, and when they are not in equal amounts, the body will be unhealthy in various ways. One ayurvedic theory asserts that each human possesses a unique combination of dosas that define that person's temperament and characteristics. Another view, also present in the ancient literature, asserts that humoral equality is identical to health, and that persons with preponderances of humors are proportionately unhealthy, and that this is not their natural temperament. In ayurveda, unlike the Sankhya philosophical system, there are twenty fundamental qualities, guṇa (Devanagari, meaning qualities) inherent in all substances. Ayurvedic theory asserts that building a healthy metabolic system, attaining good digestion, and proper excretion leads to vitality. Ayurveda also focuses on exercise, yoga, and meditation,

The practice of *panchakarma* (Devanagari) is a therapeutic way of eliminating toxic elements from the body. Eating red meat is like poisoning your blood stream; it has lots of toxins and hormones.

As early as the Mahabharata, ayurveda was called "the science of eight components" (Skt. astanga Devanagari). It is a way to also find balance, good balance, or "good trip." That is why it is so important to cleanse the whole body, mind, and soul before engaging into sacramental use of entheogens.

Now igniting the experience.

Experiencing With The Help Of Tantra

Tantra practical technique does follow below: remember always to start with small amount of entheogens. Tantra, when mixed with entheogenic substances, is like pouring high-octane gasoline into fire! Caution is advised.

The Technique:

First, understand something basic. One, if you have observed at all you must have observed that your sex energy moves with imagination. Just through imagination, your sex center starts functioning. Really, without imagination, it cannot function. Why am I emphasizing this fact? Because if imagination helps the energy to move, then you can move it upward or downward just by imagination. You cannot move your blood by imagination; you cannot do anything else in the body by imagination. But sex energy can be moved by imagination. You can change its direction. This sutra says, "Consider your essence as light rays." Think of yourself, your being, as light rays "from center up the vertebrae"—up your spine—and so rises "livingness" in you. Yoga has divided your spine into seven centers. The first is the sex center and the last is sahasrar, and between these two there are five centers. Some systems divide into nine, some into three, some into four. Division is not very meaningful; you can make your own division. Just five centers are enough to work with. The first is the sex center, the second is just behind the navel, the third is just behind the heart, the fourth is behind your two eyebrows, just in between the middle of the forehead. And the fifth, sahasrar, is just on the peak of your head. These five will do. This sutra (has similarities with mantras, see patanjali) says, "Consider yourself . . . ," which means imagine yourself—close your eyes and imagine yourself just as if you are light. This is not just imagination. In the beginning it is, but it is reality also because everything consists of light. Now science says that everything consists of electricity, and Tantra has always said that everything consists of light particles—and you also. That is why the Koran says that God is light. You are light! Imagine first that you are just light rays; then move your imagination to the sex center. Concentrate your attention there and feel that light rays are rising upward from the sex center, as if the sex center has become a source of light and light rays are moving in an upsurge—upward toward the navel center. Division is needed because it will be difficult for you to connect your sex center with the sahasrar. So smaller divisions will be of help. If you can connect, no divisions are needed. You can just drop all divisions from your sex center onward, and the energy, the life force, will rise up as light toward the sahasrar. But divisions will be more helpful because your mind can conceive of smaller fragments more easily. So just feel that the energy—just the light rays—is rising up from your sex center to your navel like a river of light. Immediately, you will feel a warmth rising in you. Soon your navel will become hot. You can feel the hotness; even others can feel that hotness. Through your imagination, the sex energy will have started to rise. When you feel that now, the second center at the navel has become a source of light, that the rays are coming and being collected there; then start to move to the heart center. As the light reaches the heart center, as the rays are coming, your heartbeat will be changed. Your breathing will become deeper, and a warmth will come to your heart. Go on upward. "Consider your essence as light rays from center to up the vertebrae, and so rises "livingness" in you.

And as you will feel warmth, just side by side, you will feel a "livingness," a new life coming to you, an inward light rising up. Sex energy has two parts: one is physical and one is psychic.

The sex energy is the psychic part of it, and the psychic part can rise. And for that psychic part, the spinal passage is used—the spinal passage and its centers. But that has to be felt. The feeling center must start functioning; only then will these techniques be of any help. Otherwise, you will go on thinking that energy is rising, but there will be no feeling (feel it). And if there is no feeling, imagination is impotent, futile. Only a feeling imagination will give you a result. We pictured sahasrar as a lotus—as a thousand-petaled lotus. Sahasrar means thousand petalled—an opening of a thousand petals. Just conceive of the lotus with a thousand petals, opened, and from every petal this light energy is moving into the cosmos. Again, this is a love act—not with nature now, but with the ultimate. Caution: Don't leave this energy anywhere. Allow it to come to the sahasrar.(why is so important the cleanser of the chakras "perineum, G-spot" as mentioned before, remember this). Whenever you do this experiment, don't leave it in the middle. You have to complete it. Take care that no one disturbs you. If you leave this energy somewhere in the middle, it can be harmful. It has to be released. So bring it to the head and feel as if your head has become an opening. But don't leave the energy somewhere in the body at some center. Someone may come and you will have some business, or some phone call will come and you will have to stop. So do it at such a time that no one will disturb you, and don't leave the energy in any center. Otherwise, that center where you leave the energy will become a wound, and you may create many mental illnesses. So be aware; otherwise don't do this. This method needs absolute privacy (like I mentioned before a couple of times), and no disturbance, and it must be done completely. The energy must come to the head, and it should be released from there. Note: Again, it is an orgasm. There are two types of orgasms: one is sexual and the other spiritual. The sexual comes from the lowest center and the spiritual from the highest center. From the highest you meet the highest and from the lowest you meet the lowest. Even while actually in the sex act, you can do this exercise; both the partners can do this. Move the energy upward, and then the sex act becomes Tantra sadhana; it becomes meditation. You will have various experiences.

When you will feel that the rays are starting to come up from the sex center, there will be various sensations at the sex center. When you start meditation, the sex center will become more sensitive, alive, excited, and in the beginning the excitement will be just the same as any sexual excitement—but only in the beginning. As your meditation becomes deeper, you will feel energy flowing up. As the energy flows, the sex center becomes silent, less excited. When the energy will really move to the sahasrar, there will be no sensation at the sex center. It will be totally still and silent. It will have become completely cool, and the warmth will have come to the head. And this is physical. When the sex center is excited, it becomes hot; you can feel that hotness, it is physical. When the energy will move, the sex center will become cooler and cooler and cooler, and the hotness will come to the head. You will feel dizzy. When the energy comes to the head, you will feel dizzy. Sometimes you may even feel nausea because for the first time energy has come to the head and your head is not acquainted with it. (You can move your head left to right, this helps release lots of stress.) It has to become tuned. So don't become afraid. Sometimes you may immediately become unconscious, but *don't be afraid*. This happens. If so much energy moves suddenly and explodes in the head, you may become unconscious. But that unconsciousness cannot remain for more than one hour. Within one hour, the energy automatically falls back or is released. You cannot remain that way for more than one hour. I say one hour, but in fact, it is exactly forty-eight minutes. It cannot be more than that. It never has been in millions of years of experiments, so don't be afraid. If you do become unconscious, it is okay. After that unconsciousness, you will feel so fresh that it is as if you have been in sleep for the first time, in the deepest sleep. Yoga calls it by a special name—yoga tandra, or yogic sleep. It is very deep; you move to your deepest center. But don't be afraid. And if your head becomes hot, it is a good sign. Release the energy. Feel as if your head is opening like a lotus flower—as if energy is being released into the cosmos. As the energy is released, you will feel a coldness coming to you. You have never felt the coldness that comes after this hotness. But do the technique completely; never do it incompletely. (Tip: in the beginning, do release the stress; in the end of the exercise, you can have also physical multiple orgasms, both partners; but when you are no longer a novice, you feel less desire to dissipate that precious energy). You can also have multiple orgasms by stimulating G-Spot, releasing tons of accumulated stress.

The Second Technique:

"Or in the spaces between, feel this as lightning." This is a very similar method with a slight difference: between one center and another; as rays are coming, you can feel it like lightning.

Just a jump of light. For some people, the second will be more suitable, and for others the first. This is why there is a modification. There are people who cannot imagine things gradually, and there are people who cannot imagine in jumps. Why do I try to address both techniques? If you can think and imagine gradually, then the first method is good. But if you try the first method and you suddenly feel that from one center the rays jump directly to the second, then don't do the first method. The second is better for you. Feel this as lightning—like a spark of light jumping from one center to the next. For those who can conceive of jumps, the second modification is best. Think of this as lightning in the sky, in the clouds, just jumping from one place to another. But choose. Try these, and choose whichever you feel is good for you.

Caution: Two or three things more about this method. With lightning, you may feel such hotness that it may seem unbearable. If you feel that, don't try it. Lightning can give you much heat. If you feel that it is unbearable, then don't try this. Then with the first method, if you are at ease, then it is good. Otherwise, with uneasiness, don't try it. Sometimes the explosion can be so great that you may become afraid of it, and once afraid, you will never be able to do it again. Then fear enters. So one has to be aware always not to become afraid of anything. If you feel that fear will come and it is too much for you, don't try it. Then the first method with light rays is best. If you feel that even with light rays too much hotness is coming to you—and it depends because people differ—then conceive of the rays as cool, imagine them as cool. Then instead of feeling warmth, you will feel a coldness with everything. That too will be effective. So you can decide; try and decide. Remember, with this technique, and with others also, if you feel very uneasy or anything unbearable, don't do it. There are other methods, and this one may not be for you. With unnecessary disturbance inside, you will create more problems than you will solve.

Note: Because of this, many centuries ago a particular yoga which we call sahaj yoga was developed. Sahaj means spontaneous, easy, natural. Always remember, sahaj. If you feel any technique spontaneously coming to you, if you feel more affinity with it, if you feel better with it—more healthy, more alive, more at home—then that is the method for you. Move with it; you can trust it. Don't create unnecessary problems. And the inner mechanism is very complex. If you do something which is too much for you, you may destroy many things. So it is better to move with something which feels harmonious to you. (Be cautious with entheogenic doses, start with small ones.) Practice brings perfection; you can practice every week if you like or even once a month is up to you. The ideal is the last choice. These exercises will promote the arousal of kundalini power and send the creative (sexual) energy to your head. This is in reality the true meaning of deal with Tantra and entheogens. If you are ready, your soul will dive into *paraatman* (supreme soul) and finally you experience God within and brings that reality to your daily life. Meanwhile, dissolving your ego, truly living enlightened, that is the meaning of taking entheogenic substances and practicing religious beliefs. Let the ocean of pure light, joy, and bliss "contaminate" your soul.

The cure is contagious.
—Dr. Eneas Lintz

Before you criticize a man, walk a mile in his shoes. That way, when you do criticize him, you'll be a mile away and have his shoes.

—Jack Handey

BIBLIOGRAPHY

Arthur Avalon: The Great Liberation Madras: Ganesh and Co., 1913. *Tantrick Texts* London: Luzac and Co., 1922 Tantraraja With a Preface by Yogi Shuddhananda Bharati. Madras: Ganesh and Co., 1954. Kulacudamani Nigana Madras: Ganesh and Co., 1956. *The Greatness of Shiva*. Madras: Ganesh and Co., 1963. (Translator). *Hymn to Kali (Karpuradi-Stotra)*. Commentary by Swami Vimalananda. Madras: Ganesh and Co., 1965

Aldous Huxley. The doors of perception, Harper & Row, 1990

Atlantis and Lemuria Frank Joseph, Edgard Cayce Readings, ARE Press, 2001

Doore, Gary
Shaman's Path: Healing, Personal Growth and Empowerment Shambhala, 1988

Drury, Nevill
The Elements of Shamanism Element, Rockport, Mass., 1993

Eliade, Mircea
Shamanism: Archaic Techniques of Ecstasy Princeton, Bollingen, 2nd printing, 1974

Phantastica Louis Lewin, M.D. 1998 Park Street Press

Goodman, Felicitas D.
    Where the Spirits Ride the Wind: Trance Journeys and Other Ecstatic Experiences Indiana University Press, 1990

Halifax, Joan
    Shamanic Voices: A Survey of Visionary Narratives E. P. Dutton, NY, 1979

Harner, Michael
    The Way of the Shaman *** Harper Collins, NY, 3rd ed., 1990

Hollow earth in the Puranas
    Dean Dominick de Lucia, TGS Services, 2000

Ingerman, Sandra
    Soul Retrieval: Mending the Fragmented Self *** Harper, San Francisco, 1991

Welcome Home: Following Your Soul's Journey Home *** Harper, San Francisco, 1993

Keeney, Bradford Shaking out the Spirits: A Psychotherapists' Entry into the Healing Mysteries of Global Shamanism Station Hill Press, 1994

Larsen, Stephen
    The Mythic Imagination: Your Quest for Meaning Through Personal Mythology Bantam, NY, 1990

Lives of the Master
   by Glenn Sander, Edgar Cayce readings, 1971, 1998
   ARE Press

Messages from the hollow earth
Dianne Robbins, Trafford, 2003

Opium for the Masses
loompanics, by Jim Hogshire, 1994

The Shaman's Doorway: Opening Imagination to Power and Myth
   Station Hill Press, Barrington, NY, 1988

Paddos, 1997 egosoft
Contributions of many people in the fields of entheogens

Psychedelic shamanism, Jim de Konne
loompanics, 1994

Palmer, Cynthia and Michael Horowitz (Eds.)
Shaman Woman, Mainline Lady Quill, NY, 1982

Plotkin, Mark J.
Tales of a Shaman's Apprentice Penguin Books, NY, 1993

Roth, Gabrielle
Maps to Ecstasy: Teachings of an Urban Shaman Notaraj, 1989

Shamanic voices
Joan Halifax, Armana, 1979

Soma the Divine Hallucinogen
David Spess

Somé, Malidoma Patrice
Of Water and the Spirit: Ritual, Magic and initiation in the Live of an African Shaman Penguin-Arkana, New York, 1994

Stevens, Jose and Lena S. Stevens
Secrets of Shamanism Avon Books, NY, 1988

Walsh, Roger N.
The Spirit of Shamanism *** Jeremy P. Tarcher/Perigee, 1990

Capra, Fritjof
The Turning Point: Science, Society and the Rising Culture Bantam, 1988

Uncommon Wisdom: Conversations with Remarkable People Bantam, 1988
    The Tao of Physics (3rd edition) *** Shambala 1991

Capra, Fritjof and David Steindl-Rast
Belonging to the Universe *** Harper, San Francisco, 1991

Fox, Matthew
Breakthrough: Meister Eckhart's Creation Spirituality Image Books,
 Doubleday, 1991

Griffiths, Bede
Universal Wisdom *** Harper San Francisco, 1994

Grof, Stanislav
The Holotropic Mind: The Three Levels of Human Consciousness
 and How They Shape Our Lives Harper, San Francisco, 1990

Kornfield, Jack
A Path with Heart Bantam, 1993

Mishlove, Jeffrey
Thinking Allowed: Conversations on the Leading Edge of
 Knowledge Council Oak Books, 1992

Swimme, Brian and Thomas Berry
The Universe Story Harper, SF, 1944

Tarnas, Richard
The Passion of the Western Mind: Understanding the Ideas That
 Have Shaped Our World View *** Ballentine, NY, 1993

The Archaic Revival
Terence Mckenna, Foreword by Tom Robbins, 1991
Harper San Francisco

The Entheogenic Evolution
Martin Ball, 2008 bear and Company

The Mystery of Manna
Dan Merkur
Psychedelic Sacrament of the Bible, Park Street Press, 2000

The Spear of Destiny
Hitler and the dark side of the power "ego"
Trevor Havenscroft, Samuel Weiser, Inc, 1982

The Road to Eleusis
R. Gordon Wasson, Albert Hofmann, Carl A. P. Ruck
North Athantic Books, 2008

Walsh, Roger N., and Frances Vaughan
Paths Beyond Ego: The Transpersonal Vision *** Jeremy P. Tarcher/
    Perigee, 1993

Wilber, Ken. The Spectrum of Consciousness *** Quest Books,
    Wheaton, Il., 1993

The Atman Project Quest Books, Wheaton, Il., 1988

Sex, Ecology, Spirituality *** Shambala, 1995

No Boundary *** Shambhala, 1979 (dimitri)

Danah Zohar and Ian Marshall
The Quantum Society William Morrow, NY, 1994

Zukov, Gary
The Dancing Wu Li Masters Bantam, NY, 1984

The Seat of the Soul Simon Schuster, 1990

Touch me There, Yvonne k Fulbright, Hunter house 2007

Friedman, Milton and Thomas S. Szasz
On Liberty and Drugs Drug Policy Foundation Press, 1992

Grof, Stanislav LSD Psychotherapy Hunter House, 1994

Lyttle, Thomas, Psychedelics Barricade, NY, 1994

McKenna, Terence
Food of the Gods *** *Bantam, 1992 (dimitri)*

Ott, Johathan
Pharmacotheon: Entheogenic Drugs, Their Plant Sources and
    History *** Natural Products, Co., 1993

Saunders, Nicholas
E for Ecstasy Biddles of Guildford, England 1993

Schultes, Richard Evans and Hofmann, AlbertPlants of the Gods
    *** McGraw Hill, 1979 (dimitri)

Shulgin, Alexander and Ann Shulgin
PHIKAL: A Chemical Love Story Transform Press, Berkeley, 1991

Wikipedia

Encyclopedia Britannica

Books from *Divine Grace A. C. Bhaktivedanta Swami Prabhupada*

Bhagavad Gita as is Macmillan 1972

Srimad Bhagavatam

Sri Caitanya caritamrta 1975

Teachings of lord Caitanya 1968

The Nectar of Devotion 1970

The Nectar of Instruction

Easy Journey to other planets 1972 (among the books that I like most)

Krsna Consciousness: The Supreme Personality of Godhead, 1970

Sri Isopanisad 1974

Among others, some of them in Portuguese language.

Books from Chico Xavier, Alan Kardec, etc.

Paul-Clément Jagot
le pouvoir de la volonte sur soi-meme, sur les austres, sur le destin (I read in Portuguese version)

Important Note:

If you are taking any MAO-inhibiting substances, avoid experience with entheogenics. caution is advised. so whatever you do with your body is your own decision, not mine.

Web sites:
   www.Shamannow.com
   www.erowid.org

www.ingramcontent.com/pod-product-compliance
Lightning Source LLC
Chambersburg PA
CBHW020741180526
45163CB00001B/308